Bun 2 Babe

Bun 2 Babe

ROUTINES AND STRATEGIES FOR NURTURING YOUR
BABY, PREGNANCY THROUGH AGE TWO: A PERSONAL
AND INFORMATIVE GUIDE FROM A MOTHER OF FOUR

~ With tips from many other amazing moms ~

Charlotte Ryan, BSc Hon, BEd, MA

ISBN-13: 9781508874942
ISBN-10: 1508874948
Library of Congress Control Number: 2015904615
CreateSpace Independent Publishing Platform
North Charleston, South Carolina

To J. C., the love of my life, and our four little miracles: T., P., E., and M.

And to Maya—it's your turn now.

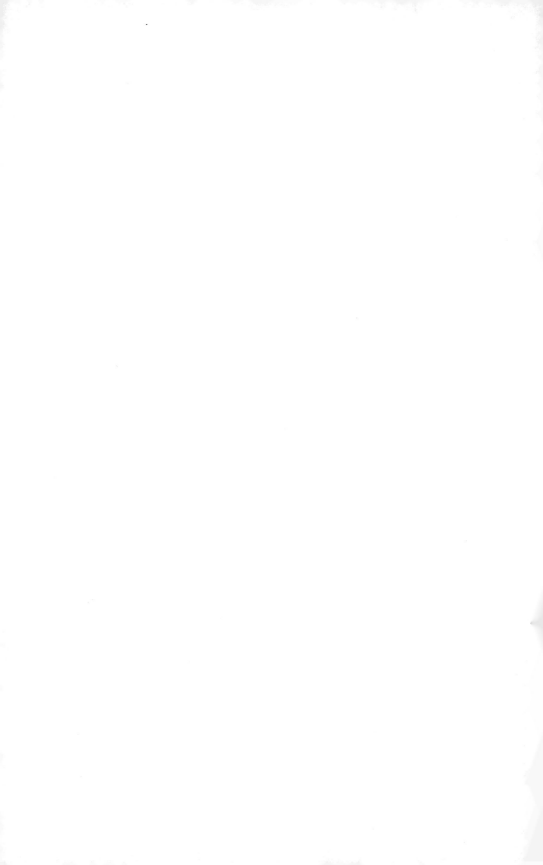

Acknowledgments

I need Mommy, or I'm going to collapse…I collapsed.
—P., AGE FIVE

I must acknowledge all my mentor-mommies and friends with whom I've talked through many problems and issues. I've incorporated much of their advice into my own strategies and have included them in this book. When you encounter a footnote with a name, that idea came from the mom mentioned.

Thank you to Tamara Adamson, Maya Castle, Brenda Cuthbertson, Gerd Griffin, Oresta Korbutiak, Carolyn Lauclan, Mary Miller, Amy Olar, Marian Orleans, Mary Anne Pangilinan, Charmayne Richards, Stacey Rinsma, Abigail Roberts[1], Samantha Rogers, Patricia Ryan, Ellen Ryan-Chan, Shalimar Santos-Comia, Lisa Simms, Lynne Strike-Teal, Alexis Taylor-Fermin, Yvette Tsang, Susan Waite, and my late grandmother May Griffin.

I would like to acknowledge all the wonderful doctors, nurses, and midwives who assisted me during my four pregnancies and births and my postpartum care. I would like to give a special thank-you to Lisa Weston and Claudette Leduc, two incredibly nurturing, caring, and knowing midwives who helped, supported, and educated me during all four pregnancies and birth experiences. They guided me when I needed them most and were always there to answer my questions and concerns.

Next, I would like to thank the incredibly helpful and knowledgeable professionals whose words I paraphrased and referenced in this book:

---

1 Name changed by request.

Dr. Lisa Doran, naturopathic doctor; Dr. Howard Berger, gynecologist; Nadia Ramprasad, physiotherapist; Dr. Karen Beal, chiropractor; and Ronald G. Morrish, parenting expert, educator and behavior consultant.

Additionally, I would like to recognize the professionals who helped me bring my book to publication. Thank-you to Rachelle Purych for her incredible illustrations, Christy Jackson of Explain the Rain Studios for overseeing art work and explainer video, Michael Kulas for the voice recording for the explainer video and Jeff Pestell and his team at Champ & Pepper for the logo. Thanks to the editors at CreateSpace: Michelle, Cynthia and June- I appreciate your thorough work and attention to detail.

I also need to express my deepest gratitude to my parents, Patricia and Terry, and my sister, Ellen, who always encouraged me in my writing or anything I set out to accomplish. A special thanks for their editing help as well. Additionally, thank-you to my father-in-law Max, for his skillful and professional final editing. And I will be forever grateful to my spectacular nanny, Rose, without whom I would never have had the time to write this book! Finally, I must thank and salute my wonderfully clever and handsome husband, J. C. Thank you, J. C., for believing in my project and helping me reach my goal!

Warning

> I don't like taking care of babies. It's
> too much work. They poo.
> —P., AGE FIVE

Babies and toddlers are needy—very needy. They need to be fed, cleaned, changed, dressed, put to bed, played with, read to, and sung to. They need their teeth brushed, shoes put on, noses wiped, hair done, faces washed, and Band-Aids applied. They need to be loved unconditionally. They need your utmost attention at all times; they take all your energy and time, and meeting their needs will consume most of your money. There are no guarantees, returns, exchanges, or warranty-protection programs. What you get back from them are immeasurable joy and love forever. Keep all of this in mind before you get one!

Foreword

Today, if the bananas fall off my pancake, I won't cry at all because I'm so excited about Christmas.

—P., Age Five

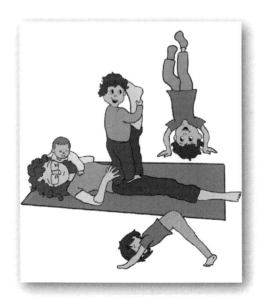

When people learn that I'm a mom to four kids, they always say that I'm crazy. Well, the truth is I *am* absolutely crazy... about my kids. Whoever knew this kind of love existed? It's the most beautiful thing. In our big family, there is so much love to go around and always someone to play with. It's certainly demanding and exhausting, but nothing could compare to the rosy, sweet love you get from these tiny little children. Yes, I have a bucket of "pet" worms/slugs and/or snails at my front door most days and a house full of helmets (hockey, ski, bike, and horseback riding times six equals *a lot* of helmets). When I go grocery shopping, I've been told that my cart looks like Santa's sleigh; I am always buying toilet paper; I spend a lot of time trimming toenails and fingernails (I have a hundred to do, including mine); and if I attempt to do yoga at home, I end up being a climbing apparatus for my kids. I've come to realize that my family is a real-life, modern version of the traditional *Family Circus* comic strip[2].

But in the midst of all of that, I get to play the best game of all: "smoochy tag" (it's my kids' favorite: we all run around, and I try to catch them and kiss them) with the best players of all: Terrek, eight; Patrick, six; Evelyn, four; and Maxwell, two. Life with kids is the best, fullest, and most wonderful life. When a stranger sees me with my four little ones on the way to the park and says sarcastically, "You got enough kids there?" I just smile and say, "Yes, thank you—the perfect amount." ☺

I have always been an overachiever in everything I do. My latest "project" and life goal is to do an incredible job of raising my children. I want to do everything I can to help my kids be the best they can be: kind, smart, healthy, caring, sensible, and loving. Just as my husband is a workaholic, working so hard to provide for our four kids, I'm a "momaholic": I work so hard to love, care for, nurture, and educate our four kids. I've tried theories out and modified them to make them work for my family. Because I have had the pleasure of trying out my strategies four times, at this point I've fine-tuned them and made them my own. I have figured out what really works.

When it comes to babies, I've tried and done it all. I have had four completely different birth experiences and four different child-care arrangements. I've tried cosleeping and crib sleeping; pureed baby foods for feeding and whole foods baby-led weaning; cloth diapers and disposable diapers, and more, more, more! During the past eight

---

2 Bil Keane, http://familycircus.com/strip-archives/

years, I have gone through a lot when it comes to babies. Now I can pass that wealth of experience on to you, the new parents.

As a parent, you're constantly learning. You are always faced with new dilemmas and interesting, annoying, worrisome, frustrating, and/or hilarious problems to solve. When I first finished writing my rough draft of this book one year ago, my dilemma of the day was what to do with the cup that fell in the toilet. Clean it or toss it? (We tossed it.) In addition to that, here's a snapshot of the problems I was working out right then with my four kids. My oldest, Terrek, was testing my patience because instead of coming when he was called, he would go in the opposite direction, investigating some bug or a speck of dirt. Patrick, my then-five-year-old, was too focused and busy to eat his snacks at school. Then when he got home from school, he was *starving* and wanted to eat everything in sight. Evelyn, my little girl, kept putting her precious blankie in her nose and getting boogers on it. Finally, my baby, Maxwell, so cute and adorable, but—watch out—he bit! Now, one year later, all those problems have been solved, and I've moved on to new ones.

Now, as I write this, the dilemma of the day is, the kids got into my husband's expensive hair product and used it *all* up giving themselves Mohawks. Maxwell's Mohawk looked more like large globs of guck smeared on the top of his head. (They attempted hairstyling with my face cream first, realized that didn't work, and then went on to the good stuff.) As we grow as a family, each individual child keeps bringing us new challenges. Currently I'm struggling with Terrek, now eight, as his behavior changes with age, testing my husband and me. He's trying to establish more independence. I want to give him more independence but at the same time keep my little boy safe. (No, you can't go to the park by yourself yet.) Patrick, now six, is going through an extremely clingy phase. He climbs me like a tree and holds on for dear life quite a lot of the time; getting him to let go is something of a feat. Evelyn, four, is in a phase where she hates underwear with a passion; she wants to wear her pajamas or her bathing suit all day to avoid wearing anything underneath. Maxwell, who's just mastered potty training, has learned that if he lies and says, "Max go poo!" even when he doesn't actually need to go, he can put off going to bed or get out of his car seat if he feels he's been sitting there too long. See? I don't have all the answers (but I do have a lot), and that is because I am still learning and problem solving as I go. This is your new life as a parent. This book shares the tips and advice that I have figured out to be effective in nurturing and caring for your newborn baby, up through the first two years. Good luck. Here you go! Embrace your baby and enjoy your own unique journey!

Disciaimer

Maxwell, don't play with Terrek's penis. You
have your own penis you can play with.
—E., AGE THREE

This book is entirely the opinion of an experienced mother of
four. It is not intended to replace medical or professional advice.
Readers are encouraged to consult their doctors, midwives,
and/or other professional caregivers for their own needs.

I have intentionally left out brand names of products mentioned
and described in this book unless it was for something very specific.
I want this book to remain a neutral and unbiased reference for new
parents. I mention a brand-name item a few times because I believe
it's the only one of its kind, and I want to increase your chances of
being able to find it. I am not affiliated with any of the brands and do
not receive any incentive to mention them. The products are honestly
things that I have used or recommend from my own experience.

Finally, please note that this book is written from the perspective
of a mother in a traditional two-parent, heterosexual marriage; however, the advice and guidance I provide are applicable to all family
situations where a new baby has come into your life.

A Note about the Music

I don't like this song…it tastes weird.

—E., Age Three

I have referred to many fantastic songs throughout this book that help me tell my story. To get the full effect I intended as I wrote this book, feel free to check out the referenced song, marked by the symbol ♪, as you read: go to iTunes (http://www.apple.com/ca/itunes/?cid=wwa-ca-kwg-music-itu), have a listen, and even buy a song if it speaks to you or brightens your day. Sometimes I'm hoping you really pay attention to the lyrics; other times the mention is a humorous add-on to my train of thought. The songs really seemed to fit the theme of the topic at hand; consider them a soundtrack to the book, adding an extra layer to the experience. I hope you enjoy it!

Table of Contents

I don't throw spoons. I'm big. I know what I'm doing.
—E., AGE THREE

Note: The chapters appear in the order of my experience for each issue or event. For you, or in your babies' lives, some topics may surface in a slightly different order. Remember, babies (and moms and dads) are not all alike. For instance, I started introducing my babies to solid foods when they were six months old, but I didn't wean them from breastfeeding until eighteen months (two and a half years for Maxwell…). I didn't return to work until my little ones were twelve months old; where you live, maternity leave policies may differ, affecting your decision. Please keep such variety in mind as you read and in referring to the time line in chapter 2.

CHAPTER 1

It All Begins

> I sat on Patrick's dinner, and Patrick
> sat on the bananas.
>
> —ME

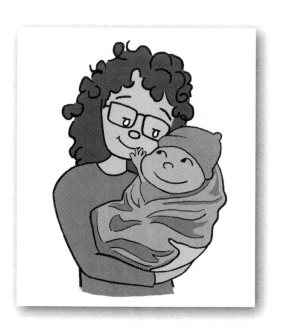

Having a baby is like falling in love. You can't stop staring at him, and you spend a lot of time holding him close in the dark. You spend every waking hour together; you are inseparable. You love to kiss him, and you find yourself completely smitten. You get to know each other more and more each day. You are developing a long-lasting, intimate bond…and he really likes your breasts—just like falling in love! It really does seem too good to be true.[3] ♪

Congratulations on getting to this place. It is the most wonderful journey. You will laugh out of pure joy and amazement, and you will cry with frustration and exhaustion. But above all, you will experience a deep love unlike anything you've ever felt before. You and your partner are not just a couple anymore. There are three of you now, and you're a family. This is real!

There is so much to learn, and you will learn it. You will find your own way. This book is a guide, based on my experience with four infants. Use what works for you and what helps you. My first baby was definitely the most challenging. I didn't know what I was doing! I had a lot to discover and a lot to figure out. By the fourth baby, it was easy. I had figured it out. While all babies are different, I developed systems, routines, and strategies. I took note of what worked for me, and now I'm sharing it with you. So here you go: get ready for your new baby! As I said, there is a lot to learn, but there is also a lot to get (see chapter 6, "The Gear").

---

3 "Can't Take My Eyes Off of You," Lauryn Hill, *The Miseducation of Lauryn Hill*, 1998, Ruffhouse Records and Columbia Records.

CHAPTER 2

The Time Line

This is a picture of Mommy. This is her head,
this is her hair, and these are her nipples.
—P., Age Four

This time line, based on my experiences, approximates the "when" of events in an infant's first two years. Please remember, again, that babies are unique people and may not follow this timetable exactly. Some events may happen earlier and some later, and that's all OK! Your baby is perfect just the way she is, and while you get to decide when she does some things, she gets to choose when she does others. Together, you and your baby will develop your own schedule. As a general reference, here is mine.

Prebirth Time Line

Gestation Period	Event
Before pregnancy:	- Take folic acid supplements (Mom and Dad[4]).
1 month P.:	- Use a home pregnancy test when you suspect you're pregnant. - Make an appointment with a family doctor to confirm pregnancy.

4 http://www.whattoexpect.com/preconception/ask-heidi/folic-acid-and-male-fertility.
aspx

- Decide if you want a midwife or an obstetrician/gynecologist to care for you during pregnancy, birth, and postpartum.
- Sign up at todaysparent.com and/or babycenter.com for regular updates on typical fetal development.
  - Note: these websites project and track your baby's physical growth and milestones by sending you relevant articles on the phases from pregnancy through childhood.

2 months P.:
- Nausea starts.
  - Mommy needs lots of rest; she'll be very tired.
  - Mommy may want to take Diclectin (available in Canada and in other countries under a different name), or vitamin B_6.[5] Ask your doctor or midwife.
  - The nausea that accompanies the first three to four months of pregnancy makes these months the most challenging to get through for many. Being sick and vomiting is so difficult to endure, especially when you still have to work and function in society. For two of my four pregnancies, I took the medication Diclectin, which your doctor or midwife can prescribe. I initially resisted medication for fear of side effects, but, for me, this drug had none, and it's considered quite safe.[6] You may feel very tired at first until your body adjusts to it, but the drug really helps fend off the debilitating nausea itself!

5 www.babycenter.com/404_does-vitamin-b6-help-relieve-morning-sickness_2519.bc
6 http://www.motherisk.org/prof/updatesDetail.jsp?content_id=940

3 months P.:	- First ultrasound.

- First ultrasound.
  - Get ready to be in awe. You will catch a glimpse inside your swelling belly and see an actual baby with tiny feet, arms, legs, fingers—everything. He or she will be wiggling and moving and may even appear to wave or suck a thumb. It's surreal. You will most likely cry.
- Blood tests.
  - Decide if you want to have genetic screening for your baby. (For my part, I decided that more information is good—the more informed you are, the better the decisions you can make, and the more prepared you will be.)
  - After twelve weeks, you can tell people about your pregnancy, as you have passed the most clinically vulnerable stage.
  - Mommy's tummy starts to swell.
  - If you're working outside the home, inform your employer of pregnancy and your intention to take maternity leave, if applicable.
  - Apply for pregnancy/parental leave.

5 months P.:
- Second ultrasound.
  - Find out Baby's gender (if you want!).
    - o As long as Baby is in an agreeable position, you can discover the gender, but if Baby is turned with bottom facing the front, the genitals may be hidden from the camera's view. (Hmph, hmph Eveyln!)
    - o Some ultrasound clinics refuse to disclose the gender of Baby. If you are eager to know the sex, then you

should ask about policy when you book your appointment.
- Feel the baby kick for the first time.
  • It feels like a bubble popping in your stomach. It may feel similar to a bubble of gas.
- Nausea starts to subside.
- Register for baby shower items.
  • Shopping is fun!

6 months P.:
- Arrange Baby's room.
- Assemble crib, changing table, etc.
- Baby moves around a lot; you'll feel kicks, stretches, and squirms.
- Take a prenatal class with your husband/ partner.
  • Note: Consider avoiding watching the birth video shown in class. I thought it was horrible, not helpful, and it just makes you nervous. I regretted seeing it.

7 months P.:
- Install the baby car seat.
  • Your local police station, fire station, or community center may run car seat clinics to teach you how to attach your seat or check that you've done it correctly. Use this free resource!
  • The above professionals often place cut pool noodles beneath bucket-style infant car seats to set them at the correct angle.

8 months P.:
- Pack a hospital bag.
- Make a birth plan.
  • Write out your wishes for caregivers: When do you want to go to the hospital? How do you hope to deal with pain?

Which jobs do you have for whom? Who do you want present for the birth?

- Check with health insurance provider about coverage for hospital room (semiprivate or private).
- You can preregister at the hospital if you'd like (not necessary, but this can save time later) and provide your health insurance information at that point.
- Strep B screening.
  - These bacteria may be present in the vagina; if they are, Mom will need an IV with antibiotics at birth so Baby will not be affected. These bacteria are very common, so even if you don't have it in the first pregnancy, you may in the next.
- Think of baby names.
- Baby begins to move less because there isn't much room to stretch out anymore.
  - Flips and somersaults turn into stretches and kicks.
- Baby turns, with head pointing down (hopefully!).
  - Baby's head needs to be pointing down (toward vagina) for a normal vaginal delivery. If Baby's head is up and his bottom is pointing down—the breech position—you may need a C-section.
  - Doctors can try some maneuvering to coax the baby into a head-down position. It's a procedure performed in the hospital by pushing on the mother's belly. (I almost had to try this with Maxwell, but to my relief, he moved headfirst—see below—a few days before my appointment.) The procedure can be uncomfortable but

worth it if you want to avoid a C-section, which is, of course, major surgery.[7]

- You can also get help from a chiropractor who specializes in prenatal care. Some manual chiropractic adjustments may affect the neurobiomechanics of the pelvis, promoting a safer and easier labor for the mom and baby.[8] I saw a chiropractor when Maxwell was in the breech position, and, after seven adjustments, he moved to the headfirst position. As my chiropractor theorized, "balancing the pelvis and taking tension out of the ligaments helps to normalize the physiology," which may encourage breech babies to move into the head-down position.[9]

Drinking raspberry leaf tea at this stage might be helpful, since it's thought to help tone the uterus in preparation for childbirth.[10]

9 months P.:
- Stop working.
- Prewash, fold, and put away baby clothes, size zero to one month/newborn.
- Put clean sheets on the crib and in the playpen.
- Set up clean baby towels near washed baby bath.
- Set up a bouncy chair in the bathroom and kitchen.
- Some moms enter a "nesting phase," where they go crazy cleaning the house.

7 http://www.babycentre.co.uk/a158/breech-birth
8 Dr. Karen Beal, chiropractor
9 Ibid.
10 Claudette Leduc and Lisa Weston, registered midwives (RMs)

(It happened to me. I remember reorganizing all my laundry room cupboards the day before I went into labor with Evelyn.)
- Baby "drops" (begins descent into the birth canal in preparation for birth.
    • This can occur anywhere from two weeks prior to the actual day of labor.
    • A quick test to know when the baby drops: See whether you can place your hand flat, under your rib cage and above your belly. If you can, then chances are the baby has dropped. If your hand still rests in a curve on your big belly, then baby likely hasn't dropped yet.
- Have baby!

Postbirth Time Line

Baby's Age   Event

0 days: - Baby is born.
                              - Breastfeeding starts.
                              - Name the baby.
                              - Bank your baby's cord blood.
                                  • Cord blood banking is like a form of health insurance for your family. These cells can help with medical treatments for certain diseases if ever your baby, a sibling, or you are faced with such an illness later in life.[11]
                              - Obtain the statement of live birth from the hospital (in Canada) or fill out hospital-provided forms and mail away for the birth certificate (United States).[12]

11 www.todaysparent.com/pregnancy/giving-birth/canadas-cord-blood-system/
12 http://www.immihelp.com/nri/birthcertificate.html

2 to 3 days:	- Return home from hospital. - Mom's milk comes in. - Register online for birth certificate, Baby's SIN card, and health card (Canada), or apply for a social security card and add your child to your health insurance policy (United States).[13] - Apply for employment insurance (Canada). - Set up an e-mail account for the baby. • We did this for all our kids—to capture their moods, recount funny events, and send photos and videos. You can document their babyhood and childhood for them so they will always have this record to treasure, and so will you!
5 to 6 weeks:	- Mom's stiches (if any) dissolve, or she has to have them removed.

6 weeks:	- Baby starts to smile.
	- Baby starts to make eye contact.
	- Mom's body feels better.
	- Mom's postpartum bleeding stops.
	- Mom may resume sexual relations with Dad.
	- Mom can have baths and go swimming again (after any stitches are removed).
	  • Final visit with midwife.
	- Set up a bank account for your baby.
	- Set up an RESP for your baby (Canada).
	- Get life insurance.
	- Write or update your will.
	  • You must have heard that having kids is expensive…very true.

13 http://www.immihelp.com/nri/documents-after-childbirth-in-usa.html

2 months:

- First set of vaccinations for Baby.
  - In recent years, some questionable research has suggested that routine infant and childhood vaccinations cause serious negative side effects, even alleging a connection with autism. Scientists have debunked these claims as false.[14] Modern medicine and public health really have come a long way from prevaccination days. Vaccinations are important, and the diseases they help prevent are deadly. While no one likes putting foreign substances into their pure, clean little baby, it is a much better option than your baby contracting (or spreading) any of the terrible illnesses that are easily preventable with a vaccine. It hurts, and Baby cries. Nurse your baby, and she will feel better. Vaccinations are a small price to pay for a lifetime of immunity to scary viruses.
- Baby starts to hold up his head.
- Baby starts to suck on her hands.
- Baby starts sleeping for longer stretches at night.
  - Don't get too excited, as this is temporary. When babies start growing more, they will begin needing to nurse again in the wee hours. Enjoy this temporary break in night feeding for the short time it lasts! ☺

3 months:

- Baby is holding up his head with more strength.
- Baby begins to giggle.

14 http://www.cdc.gov/vaccinesafety/concerns/autism/

- Start tummy time with Baby.
  - Tummy time is just putting your baby facedown on her abdomen for short periods. (Increase the duration, as she gets stronger and more comfortable in the position. When she's squawking and her face is stuck in the blanket, she's had enough.) Soon she will begin to hold up her head in this posture and strengthen her arms, eventually progressing to rolling, wriggling, and crawling.
- Introduce a baby gym.
  - A baby gym is just a mat with toys dangling overhead. Baby can't actually play with them yet, but he will enjoy staring at them and, soon, reaching for them (then grabbing and pulling, eating, and eventually throwing them).
- Look into and set up childcare for when Mom goes back to work, as wait lists can be long.
- If formula-feeding, it may be time to transition to the nipple that has the next flow speed.
- You may now use the top rack of the dishwasher to sterilize bottles.
  - Prior to this age, bottles must be sterilized by boiling.

4 months:
- Second set of vaccinations for Baby.
- Baby starts to grab for dangling toys and attempts to bring them to her mouth to suck on them.
- Baby rolls over.

- Baby starts biting while breastfeeding.
  - Don't panic; this is usually temporary.
- Start baby sign language.
  - Note: Baby will not respond yet! Starting to sign to your baby now is really for your own training; your baby will catch on later. Read more about this wonderful strategy below and in chapter 25.
- Transition the baby from bassinet in parents' room to crib in his own room.
  - Four months is the optimal age to do this because babies are too young to notice. At five months and older, the baby is well aware of the separation and may cause a fuss.
- Baby begins playing in exerciser seat.
- Baby begins jumping in baby jumper.
  - For this activity, the baby needs to be strong enough to hold her head up.
  - My boys all loved jumping like crazy, and it was quite hilarious. My daughter wasn't interested in jumping—she just hung there most of the time.
- Baby may begin to "make strange" (cry around new people and shy away).
- Baby begins teething and therefore drooling (excessively—bibs required!).

5 months:
- Baby rolls over.
- Baby experiments with sounds: squeals, screams, giggles, raspberries, high-pitched calls, and soft coos.
- Baby begins to sit up.
  - My babies first sat up at between five and eight months. I found that the chubbier they were, the later it happened.

- Remember to use your nursing pillow to support Baby while he is learning to sit up. Place nursing pillow behind Baby, so it curves closely to either side of him. If he falls backwards or to either side, he'll land softly and safely on the pillow.
- Mom gets period back.
  - Menstruation can resume anytime from three to fourteen months postpartum (according to the moms I have talked to). Frequent breastfeeding can delay the return of the monthly visitor.

6 months:
- Start giving baby bottle or sippy cup of breast milk; continue to breastfeed on demand.
- Baby is teething and loves to bite on everything: fingers, toys, and even Mommy's chin.
- Introduce solid foods.
  - Really work on the sign language when feeding the baby. This is the perfect opportunity to learn *eat*, *drink*, *more*, and *done*.
- It's hilarious to watch Baby giggle and laugh while you pretend to eat her neck and tummy.
- Baby can start to have sips of water from a cup (fun!).
- If bottle-feeding, it's time to switch to next nipple flow speed.

7 months:
- Baby goes through a "beat up Mommy" phase sometime around now—he bites, pinches the skin hard by squeezing with his

tiny fists and digging into your flesh with his sharp little fingernails, and he yanks hair! It's a good thing he's so cute! Not to worry, this phase will pass quickly. Be firm, kind and consistent with your tone, e.g., "no biting, we touch gently."

- Babyproof your house now (if you haven't already done so.)

8 months:

- Baby loves to squirm around on the floor.
  - Let Baby do this a lot; it's training him to crawl.
- Baby starts to crawl.
  - My babies all started to crawl between seven and nine months.
  - Babies often crawl backward first.
  - Sometimes crawling can look weird. Two out of my four babies crawled normally. Terrek crawled with one straight leg and one bent leg. Maxwell didn't crawl regularly at first; for two months, he pulled himself along on his belly with his elbows! My nephews did a weird "crawl" on their backs with their heads! I know other babies who didn't crawl but instead scooted along on their bums in a seated position. Your baby will figure out her own way to move around.
- Baby can burp by himself.
- Baby babbles a lot!
  - "Mamamama, dadadadada, nananana, babababa."
- Baby is teething like crazy.
  - Baby bites and eats everything she can get her hands on!

- The drooling phase will likely end sometime soon.
  - My kids all ceased their massive drooling between seven and twelve months.
- Transition from bucket-style infant car seat to larger three-in-one car seat. Baby remains rear-facing.

9 months:
- Sleep train baby.
- Baby claps his hands!
- Baby starts making some simple signs, like *done*, *more*, and *milk*.
- Baby loves to smile and wave at herself in the mirror.
- Baby begins the "getting into everything" phase.
- Baby learns to wave hi and bye-bye.
- Baby pulls self to a standing position.

10 months:
- Baby starts to "cruise" (hangs on to furniture and walks).
- Baby can get comfortable with bottle and/or sippy cup.
- Baby starts to walk while holding on to a parent's hands.
- Baby starts to make more signs, like *drink* and *change*.

11 months:
- Phase out dream feed (nursing while Baby is asleep or half-asleep).
- Phase out pumping.
- Baby stands, unassisted.
- Baby starts dancing.
- Baby plays peekaboo and finds it absolutely hilarious.

- Baby is constantly into everything!
  - For example, opening drawers and emptying contents, playing in the toilet, climbing stairs, pulling the safety plugs out of electrical sockets, and/or eating any speck to be found on the floor.
  - Some babies investigate more than do others. Maxwell seems to get himself into so much more mischief than my other three combined!

11½ months:
- Start transition to childcare—visit day care or have meetings with nanny to get Baby used to new caregiver(s).
- Baby says first word, such as "mama" or "ball."

12 months:
- Begin first phase of weaning.
- More vaccinations.
- Baby learns to walk.
- Baby learns to say more words.
- Baby learns to nod for yes and shake head for no.
- Baby learns own additional signs for expressions like *shhh* and *where*.
- Baby can have time-outs now (only for a minute).
- Begin brushing Baby's teeth with infant toothpaste.
- Mom goes back to work. (Remember, this is my time line; legally mandated employer maternity leave varies significantly among countries, anywhere from three months in the United States[15] to one

---

15 http://www.dol.gov/whd/fmla/

year in Canada and England[16] to 420 days in Sweden.[17]

- Baby starts enjoying TV, such as Elmo (always a favorite).
- Baby's vocabulary increases.
- Teach Baby manners signs: *sorry*, *please*, and *thank-you*.
- Baby learns how to feed self with baby spoon and baby fork.
- Consider the timing for transitioning from a rear-facing to a forward-facing car seat. Ontario law permits the switch any time after Baby weighs twenty pounds;[18],[19] however, experts say the longer you can leave your baby rear-facing, the safer he remains. Transport Canada suggests waiting until at least age two.[20],[21] In Sweden, where many children remain rear-facing passengers until they're four years old, rates of child injury and death from car accidents are reportedly extremely low.[22]

15 months: - More vaccinations.

---

16 https://www.gov.uk/maternity-pay-leave/leave

17 http://www.huffingtonpost.ca/2012/05/22/maternity-leaves-around-the-world_n_1536120.html

18 http://www.mto.gov.on.ca/english/faq/safety.shtml#passenger

19 http://www.theglobeandmail.com/globe-drive/culture/commuting/how-long-should-my-baby-be-in-a-rear-facing-car-seat/article5958964/

20 http://www.healthychildren.org/English/safety-prevention/on-the-go/Pages/Car-Safety-Seats-Information-for-Families.aspx

21 http://www.theglobeandmail.com/globe-drive/culture/commuting/how-long-should-my-baby-be-in-a-rear-facing-car-seat/article5958964/

22 Ibid.

18 months:	- Finish weaning baby from breastfeeding (this cutoff is flexible—make it suit you both).
	- Final infant vaccinations.
	- Baby begins to speak in short, grammatically incorrect sentences.
	- Baby gets more and more confident with walking.
	- Baby learns to run.

2 years:
- The terrible twos—get ready, be prepared. On second thought, nothing can prepare you! The terrible twos are hard. Yes, your baby turns into a stubborn and emotional toddler who has tantrums. It's a hard age, but an amazing age, too—your child is figuring out who she is.
- Transition to big bed—(you can postpone this if you keep baby in a sleep bag, so he can't climb out of the crib).
- The "why" phase begins. "Why? How come? Why? Why, Mommy?"

2 to 2½ years:
- Potty training.
- Transition from crib to big kid bed.
- Baby's first hair cut
  • Be sure to save a lock of Baby's hair for the baby book.
  • Note: the age for the first hair cut will vary greatly from child to child. My kids were all around age two when we first cut their hair.
- Note: I notice the most change between ages two and three. Your toddler will change from a baby to a small child during this one year!

CHAPTER 3

Pregnancy

When I was in your tummy, how
did you know my name?
—T., Age Four

This is the most magical time. There is a little miracle growing inside you, a real human being. It's wonderful and beautiful… and it sucks. I have to be honest; being pregnant is not easy. It's hard on your body. You will most likely feel sick, tired, uncomfortable, and in pain. The baby will be sucking your energy and your nutrients. Your baby will grow and stretch your stomach beyond recognition (good-bye forever, cute, flat tummy). Will it be worth it? Yes, it will.

Through all the bodily issues that you may encounter throughout your pregnancy (some women don't get sick at all—lucky ducks) comes a deep understanding that something truly incredible is taking place within. From the astonishing change in your body when your belly starts to swell to feeling the baby kick for the first time, this understanding makes all the aches and pains bearable, even enjoyable. The pregnancy glow is a real thing. Look at a pregnant woman; she is radiant in part because of the deep happiness coming from within. Her body knows it's doing something miraculous. That's why you should take the following descriptions of possible discomforts during pregnancy with a grain of salt. The ouches are a small price to pay for such an unbelievable reward. For now, when you're not vomiting, you're a shiny, happy person![23] ♪

I could always sense I was pregnant before the home test told me so, because I could feel it in my breasts. They became more sensitive. I felt more aware of them. My breasts were my internal alarm system: Attention! You are pregnant! Get ready—here we go! (Peeing all the time starts very early as well.)

The first trimester was always the hardest for me. The constant nausea was difficult to endure. Bad smells (composting or recycling bin, inside the dishwasher, sour milk) would make me vomit, and my gag reflex was on high alert. Brushing my teeth or a hair in my mouth would set it off. (Bubblegum and cinnamon were the only toothpaste flavors I could sort of tolerate—experiment to find yours.) Continuing to work was difficult when I was fighting the urge to run to the garbage can.

When you have other children at home, it's especially hard to be sick all the time. Your kids won't let you lie on the couch, and it is very disturbing to them when their mother throws up. (They try to watch, and they get in the way. My daughter, Evelyn, then one-and-a-half, said "uh-oh" when she saw me vomit for the first time. My sons asked, "Mommy, what are you doing? You threw up? Why did you do that?") In my third and fourth pregnancies, I found relief with Diclectin (available in Canada, and other countries under different names), a medication your doctor or midwife can prescribe for morning sickness (which, by the way, should be called all-day sickness). At first, you may feel even more tired than you already were, but once your body adapts, you feel better. *What a relief!* It's considered completely safe for use in pregnancy.[24] If you are concerned about safety or effects, ask your doctor or midwife.

Other measures can also get you through the nausea. I didn't know it while pregnant, but while researching for this book I learned that taking vitamin B_6 could have effects similar to the medication,

---

23 "Shiny Happy People," R.E.M., album: *Out of Time*, 1991, Warner Bros.

24 http://www.motherisk.org/prof/updatesDetail.jsp?content_id=940

just be sure to take the recommended dosage.[25] For me, a sip of ginger ale was a lifesaver, as was the smell of fresh lemon;[26] carry around a slice in a zip-lock bag for instant relief. Having constant access to snacks is a must; I noticed my nausea was at its worst when I was hungry. Hard candies, dry cereal, and crackers also helped me make it through the yucky sick feeling throughout the day.

Get ready to be exhausted. While the baby is growing in you, your body is using up a great deal of energy to build the little guy/gal. You will feel so sleepy, especially in the first and third trimesters. I know this is probably advice you've heard before, but that's because it truly is worth listening to: *Rest now!* No matter how many people attempt to warn you, you have no idea how tired you will be when the baby comes. When you are feeding, changing, burping, and rocking a newborn around the clock, you will be more exhausted than you've ever been. You will be in a fog. So go to sleep now; it's bedtime!

Aches and pains vary from person to person as pregnancies progress, though there seems to be a direct relationship between the size of your belly and the size of your complaints! In my third trimester, heartburn became a problem. It's not just an annoyance; it really hurts. Eating almonds helps,[27] as do antacids and vanilla ice cream (yum!), and my midwives recommended papaya enzymes.[28] I also suffered butt cramps in each pregnancy, for some reason more often at night. The only remedy was a good massage—my husband or a good friend (thanks, Lynne!) repeatedly punching the fleshy part of my bottom.

Sleep time becomes uncomfortable, so stock up on lots of pillows to support your belly, legs, and back. Falling asleep also becomes hard, even though you are exhausted, and after you finally do drift off, you may wake up in the night, unable to sleep again. I found meditation helped—telling the brain, "You are in your bed. You are sleepy; you are relaxed. You are in your bed…"

---

25 www.babycenter.com/404_does-vitamin-b6-help-relieve-morning-sickness_2519.bc

26 Shalimar Santos-Comia, RN and mom

27 Claudette Leduc, RM, and Lisa Weston, RM

28 Ibid

Some women also suffer back pain, swollen feet and legs, varicose veins, stretch marks, frequent urination, tight sensation over the belly, sore breasts, hip pain…and the list goes on.

The good news about being pregnant, besides the obvious *good news,* is that you now have an excuse for confused, absent-minded, spacy, or otherwise embarrassing lapses in focus. I once tried opening the front door to my house with the clicker for my car keys and couldn't figure out why it wasn't working. Forgetting names, putting things back in the completely wrong place, and telling your husband to have a good bath at work can now be attributed to something called "pregnancy brain." Expectant moms have all "had" it and joked about it, but, apparently, it's a real phenomenon.[29] Now is the time for your sense of humor! You and everyone around you can get a chuckle from this new source of entertainment.

During pregnancy, it is essential to take maternity multivitamins with folic acid. Folic acid is, actually, important even before you conceive. I also took essential fatty acids/fish oil supplements. Look for a brand that is safe for pregnancy and free of mercury, which fish oils can contain. I used Efanatal, but apparently, it isn't available anymore.

Pregnancy is also the time to eat! You get to eat for you and for your growing baby—bonus! Food, food, and more food—who doesn't love food? Oh, how much fun eating can be…except when all food seems disgusting. It may be hard to imagine, but in the first trimester, food can be incredibly unappetizing as the nausea caused by raging pregnancy hormones kicks in. The first trimester is when you know you need to eat but ironically sometimes it feels as if you're force-feeding yourself.

Food aversions, also known as being repulsed by particular foods, are very common at this stage. Sometimes I found only one or two things I could eat that would not make me want to vomit—leading to highly specific cravings. Here is when the classic scenario of the poor, disheveled husband driving around looking for pickles in the middle of the night becomes a reality. There is some truth to this cliché! My loving husband always went out of his way to help fulfill my

---

29 http://www.todaysparent.com/family/family-health/mommy-brain/

irrational dietary urges. The satisfaction of finally enjoying the one and only food you can imagine having any desire for is spectacular. During my pregnancies, I craved (at various times) cheese and yogurt, citrus fruits, shredded lettuce, veggie burgers, subs, dill pickles, and french fries. I could not stand barbecued chicken smells, chickpeas and beans (for my first two pregnancies), and whole bananas. (Bananas cut into pieces were perfectly acceptable.) There is no rhyme or reason for the yearnings and aversions. It may be your baby saying, "I want this!" and "I don't want that!" If you listen to this little voice, eating will be much easier. And if your husband/partner is sweet enough to listen to this voice, you both will be happier!

So yes, pregnancy can be difficult to endure, and it feels like it will go on forever, especially near the end. You will feel uncomfortable and huge! Even tying your shoes is quite a challenge—let alone putting on your pants. But then it is over, and you may come to miss the wondrous sensation of the little life moving and kicking inside. So throughout the physical misery and uncontrollable urges, remember to try to treasure this beautiful, magical, physically draining time.

Unfortunately, pregnancy does things to your body that mark it forever. It's best to prepare yourself mentally now. Try to put a positive spin on these alterations to your young and firm physique. Mothers learn to laugh about these changes in a kind of sad, sarcastic way, remembering what our bodies were like before. Stretch marks will most probably inscribe your tummy, breasts, and legs; think of them as little blue-and-red crayon scribbles of love from your child. Your breasts will be saggy and droopy after you're finished with breastfeeding. They may resemble old socks. Think of these as adorable, snuggly, well-loved stuffed animals to cuddle with at night. Your nipples will likely point at the floor instead of straight ahead. Think of that as a refreshing change from headlights to flashlights shining down in the dark so you don't stub your toe on a pile of toys on the floor. Your belly button may change permanently from a cute little "innie" with a teenage piercing scar to a warped "outie" that looks like a nose. Don't worry: your new navel will provide a solution to the argument of which child gets to push the button in the elevator. One gets to do that, and the other gets to push "the squishy button on Mommy's tummy." Now everyone's happy. Your flat, toned belly will likely become a squishy, roly-poly belly with no muscles left in it because they were stretched out, with extra skin hanging like a big deflated balloon. Alas, that can actually come in handy if you ever need a stress ball to squeeze because your kids are driving you crazy; now you've got one conveniently with you all the time, and it's pretty difficult to lose. You're so pregnant![30] ♪

While it is true that your body will never quite be the same, neither will your heart and soul, which are forever changed—oh so much for the better. My oldest son, Terrek, told me when he was three, "Mommy, I love you harder than anything." I feel that way. It's intense and it's astounding. I love my kids so much that it hurts—so much, that all the damage and all the changes to my body don't matter at all.

---

30 "I'm So Pregnant," Iggy Azalea "Fancy" Parody, written and produced by What's Up, Moms, featuring Meg, vocals by Alyssa, rapping by Betsy, 2014. See https://www.youtube.com/watch?v=eVuittFyM34

Pregnancy Dos and Don'ts

Some rituals, habits, and activities are big no-no's during pregnancy; others are perfectly fine, even encouraged. Here is a table to help keep it all straight.

PRENANCY DO'S AND DON'TS

DO'S

☑ Talk, read, and sing to Baby.

☑ Have partner talk, read, and sing to Baby (good for Baby to know Dad's voice).

☑ Rub and pat your growing tummy.

☑ Continue an exercise program that you are used to, if there is no risk of falling.

☑ Intimacy with your partner may be continued

☑ Eat a wide variety of healthy foods.

☑ Listen to your cravings!

☑ Drink lots of water.

☑ Rest and get plenty of sleep.

☑ Find ways to relax.

☑ Continue with regular dental cleanings (just beware of sensitive gag reflex).

☑ Spend quality time with partner.

☑ Suck on candy to help curb nausea.

☑ Snack often.

☑ Take deep breaths.

DON'TS

☒ Take hot baths (Baby can get overheated).
☒ Do exercises where you turn your abdomen (i.e., yoga spinal twists).
☒ Do inversions (yoga headstands) in the first trimester.
☒ Bike, ski, skate, Rollerblade (any sport with a risk of falling is out of the question).
☒ Engage in heavy lifting.
☒ Start a new exercise program.
☒ Ride a roller coaster.
☒ Eat unpasteurized cheese (i.e., goat, sheep, feta, brie).
☒ Eat undercooked meat.
☒ Eat raw fish (i.e., sashimi/sushi).
☒ Consume much caffeine.
☒ Have any X-rays (dental or body).
☒ Stand too close to the microwave.
☒ Drink alcohol.
☒ Smoke anything (why would you do that to your beautiful body anyway?).
☒ Take medications (unless OK'd by your doctor or midwife).
☒ Take herbal remedies or drink herbal teas (unless OK'd by your doctor or midwife).
☒ Breathe in chemicals or fumes (i.e., house paint, cleaning chemicals).
☒ Pump gas.
☒ Consume artificial sweeteners or other questionable chemical food additives.
☒ Eat foods that have been heated in plastic.
☒ Garden (a parasite that may be present in the soil could cause birth defects, toxoplasmosis).
☒ Change kitty litter (same reason as above).
☒ Worry or stress too much (the baby feels what you feel).

Note: If you are unsure of whether any food or activity is safe for you or your baby during pregnancy, call the Motherisk Helpline at 1-877-439-2744. http://www.motherisk.org/women/index.jsp

A Few Notes about Fetal Movement

After five months or so, you will be feeling your baby moving regularly. You may be advised to count the kicks each day. For some reason, I never did that, but I got used to my baby moving frequently, and I could tell when he/she was sleeping because he/she would be still. If ever worried that I hadn't felt the baby move in a while, I would go to a quiet place, put my hand on my belly, and just relax. (It is preferable to lie down if possible.) I would talk to the baby and ask the baby to move to reassure me that he/she was OK. That may sound strange, but it worked every time.

Nearer the due date, the baby's movements will change. Don't be alarmed if you don't feel her moving around as much; as she grows (around the eighth month), there's probably just no more room in your belly. She is feeling squished! She'll likely also switch from somersaults and flips to poking elbows and kicks. You may feel her move into the optimal birth position, head-down and facing your back. Watch your belly ripple, and touch your baby's foot on the other side of your skin. Your baby is not that far away now...soon you will be seeing and feeling her move in your arms. It's amazing.

CHAPTER 4

Miscarriage

Please do not read unless you have experienced a miscarriage.

A miscarriage is a devastating loss. The hopes and excitement of pregnancy—the dreams and name ideas, all of it—sadly disappears, and you are left with an emptiness and grief. It really feels like the world is over, and it's hard to imagine going on with your life. But please know, time really does heal everything, and you will move forward.

I have four wonderful and healthy children now, but I did have five pregnancies. My very first pregnancy ended with a miscarriage. Looking back on that is easier now. But at the time, I was inconsolable. It was probably the saddest moment in my life. But I healed, as will you. I thought to myself, "These things happen for a reason, that baby just wasn't meant to be…"

I've always dreamed of being a mother! I was a nurturer by instinct; it was just in me. After many years of school and a few years of working as a teacher, I became pregnant. My husband and I were overjoyed. We began thinking about baby names and wondering whether the baby would be a girl or a boy. I started talking to my baby, touching my belly with awe and fascination, wondering who was growing inside. I noticed changes in my body. My breasts were fuller and more sensitive. We told the grandparents, aunts, and uncles, and the entire family was excited about the arrival of our newest member.

I started bleeding somewhere around the eighth week. It was just spotting at first. After a few days, the bleeding became heavier, and I started having mild cramps. I saw my doctor, and she sent me for an ultrasound. My husband and I looked at the tiny dot on the screen with hope. The technician showed us the beating heart. Everything looked fine. The next day, the bleeding became very heavy, and I began to get severe cramps. I spoke to my baby, willing it to be OK. My husband took me to the emergency room that night; I was still bleeding and in agony, both emotionally and physically. We spent the night in the ER. I lost the baby. I felt it fall out of me in a little ball of blood. I don't think I've ever cried so much.

After the miscarriage, I felt an indescribable hollowness in my body. I felt like I had lost something from inside my heart. I cried and cried for a long time. Family and close friends tried to console me and to reassure me, but nothing anybody said helped—except for one thing.

The one remark that did let me feel a small glimmer of hope and peace was something my husband said: "That wasn't your baby. One day you're going to have children, and the children you are going to have wouldn't be if you had had this one." And you know something? He was right. If I had carried that baby to full term, then circumstances in my life would have changed, and the children I have now would have been different. I guess I'm saying that I feel that the four children I have now were meant to be. They are perfect in their own ways. I was waiting for them.

Miscarriages are quite common. Approximately 15 to 20 percent of pregnancies end in miscarriage.[31] It's just not common knowledge, because nobody enjoys talking about it. Miscarriages happen for many reasons: incorrect makeup of fetal chromosomes, smoking, maternal obesity, a problem with the mother's reproductive organs, infection, environmental toxins, and more.[32] I imagine that perhaps the mother's body on some level is instinctively aware something is wrong with the

31 http://www.nlm.nih.gov/medlineplus/ency/article/001488.htm
32 Ibid.

fetus, and knows it needs to let the baby go. Whatever the reason, a miscarriage is still the same sad loss.

It's important to acknowledge the loss you feel and allow yourself to grieve. Others may not understand, as they did not have the connection to the unborn baby that you did. Good hard hugs from loved ones help. Cry on their shoulders. Let them help you share your grief. Slowly, over time, you will start feeling better. One day you will be able to look back and bear to remember. There are sunny days ahead.

Keeping yourself busy and setting new goals are the best ways to begin to heal. You may want to start trying for another baby right away (or as soon as your doctor gives you the go-ahead) to let yourself feel happy and hopeful for the next possibility of new life.

For me, that wasn't an option. The doctors found a cyst on my ovary during the ultrasounds, so I had to delay pregnancy and have surgery. Thankfully, the cyst was benign. The assessment, surgery, and postoperative healing took about a year. In another year, I was pregnant again. This time, it was meant to be.

If you are unable to get pregnant again now, for whatever reason, it's still important to be active and busy and set your sights ahead. During the year following my miscarriage, I found many pursuits to focus on. I finished my master's thesis; I wrote a children's novel; I spent lots of time with my dog Jasper and my cuddly cats, Chloe and Miles. I watched movies, went out to fancy dinners with friends, and enjoyed the outdoors, walking by the lake and on nature trails with the dog. I took dance lessons with my husband and learned the tango and the cha-cha. Such distractions may feel forced at the beginning, but I found that, with time, they brought joy, and I began to feel like myself again. You will, too.

Experiencing miscarriage is traumatic and emotional. I'm so sorry for your loss. I feel your heartache and sorrow. Please know you will heal. Things happen for a reason. That was not your baby. Hopefully you will have children one day. Don't give up! Everyone has her own path. Hopefully you will become pregnant again. Maybe you're meant to rescue a beautiful child through adoption, or possibly fertility treatment or surrogacy is what you need to pursue. Your children will find you when they are meant to. Believe me, they are worth waiting for.

CHAPTER 5

New Baby, New Lifestyle: Prepare for a Change

> Maxwell stole the butter and messed around
> with it when you were in the bathroom.
> —J. C., AGE THIRTY-EIGHT

When you are waiting for a new baby, it is important to come to grips with the fact that your lifestyle is about to change drastically. You may not really understand just how different it will be. It is a good idea to mentally prepare; let me shed some light on this topic.

Change #1: Gym Memberships

I am a yogi. I love yoga, and before having children, I did yoga three to five times a week at my local studio. I was still doing serious yoga when I was nine months pregnant with my first baby. I put a hold on my gym membership just before giving birth, thinking I'd be back in a few months. I never went back. Once my baby was born, and I was healed, I couldn't leave my baby to go to the gym. I was breastfeeding and totally connected. I didn't have a babysitter, my parents and in-laws lived too far away to stand in, and my husband worked long hours. I had the job of being with my baby constantly, and with my baby was where I wanted to be. (Many gyms offer day care on-site, which could be an option for you). Finally, now, after eight years of attempting to do yoga at home (with children climbing all over me), I have returned to doing yoga at a studio. It feels great to be back, but I don't have the freedom of going as often as I did before. I have the huge responsibility of little people who miss me all day when I'm at work (and I miss them just as much!) and depend on me for their many needs. Now I go once or twice a week, if I'm lucky!

Change #2: Travel

Traveling with a baby and young children is difficult. They cry on planes, and it's hard for them to sit still. They don't like long car rides, because they are strapped into their little car seats for hours on end, and so they cry (a lot). Besides the crying, there is the huge luggage problem. With a baby comes lots of gear. You need the stroller, the bottles and the baby food, the breast pump, diapers, extra clothes, baby seat, baby toys, and so forth. Packing it all up and lugging it around is a pain. It is even more of a pain if you get somewhere and realize you have forgotten something essential (diapers, anyone?). (Once, a new mother approached me, asking if she might borrow a diaper, as she forgot hers at home. Unfortunately for the both of us, I also forgot my diapers that day). If you are traveling and the baby is sick, that's another game changer.

So traveling just isn't the same. You can't just pick up and go. If you are brave enough to venture out on a family vacation, please note: it is much easier when babies are younger than six months. When they're that little you don't have to pack up baby food, as they're still only on breast milk or formula, and they haven't started crawling or walking, so they're still content to be held and trucked around in their car seat. And although they may cry or squawk quite loudly, they still sleep a lot.

TRAVEL TIPS WITH BABIES

- ☑ Breast- or bottle-feed Baby during airplane takeoff and landing to help him pop his ears by swallowing.
- ☑ Bring a baby sling that rests on your hip to keep hands free for luggage. The sling also holds baby close in flight so your arms can rest a bit.
- ☑ Pack more than you need, because you will always run out of something.
- ☑ Use stroller clips to attach extra bags to the stroller so you don't have to carry as much.

Change #3: Pause for Theater and Movies

The theater is no place for a baby. I booked tickets for the play *I Love Lucy* when Maxwell was a few months old. At that age, he was quiet, slept a lot, and was quite content to suckle silently on my breast. I was exclusively breastfeeding, so I couldn't leave him at home with my parents while they were watching my other kids. I knew it might not work out, but I grew up loving the TV show, and when I heard the stage version was coming to Toronto, I really, really wanted to see it. Unfortunately, Maxwell himself changed "stages" between the time I purchased the tickets and when it was time to see the play. By then, at close to five months old, he was going through a phase where he would randomly screech at the top of his lungs. I only saw the opening number. My husband, my vocal baby, and I spent the duration of the musical in the lobby, watching the show from an outdated fuzzy TV. I'd excused us from the auditorium before the glaring usher could even ask, not wanting to ruin the lovely viewing experience for everyone else. To compound the bummer that was now my theater experience, I'd had to pay the full adult price for Maxwell's ticket (theater policy) even though he'd be sitting on my lap and not taking up an extra seat.

Movies are no better; they are **too loud**. I tried taking baby Evelyn to a kids' film with my husband and our boys. This time my child's volume was not the problem; it was the surround sound. I quickly became aware, more than ever before, of just how loud big-screen car racing and beating music could be. Even with cotton balls in my baby's ears, she cried and cried. I spent the rest of the movie run-time rocking her in the lobby. Other times, I've tried bringing my toddlers once they were old enough not to mind the noise, but they wound up losing interest and wouldn't sit still for long. So once again, to avoid disturbing others, we ended up walking around in the lobby.

Many movie theatres schedule special screening times for parents, toddlers and/or young babies during which the volume is turned down and the lights kept dim. You're sitting among other parents, so they mind less if your baby is causing a ruckus; their baby is likely about to cause one, too. Stick to these showings, or skip the movies altogether and wait for home video…Netflix, anyone?

Change #4: Diet and Drink

While doctors say to avoid certain foods in pregnancy (see chapter 3) such as soft cheese and raw fish, I gave these up when I was breast-feeding, too (I am supercautious—just that kind of mom). Because I had four babies back to back, I was on a sashimi/sushi-strike for eight years, basically saying sayonara to my favorite treat for a long time. I settled for cooked versions such as California rolls (no roe) and dragon rolls (avocado and tempura shrimp), but it was such a yummy and special treat to start eating real sashimi/sushi again!

Drinking alcohol is definitely off the table during both pregnancy and breastfeeding. Whatever you put into your body goes right into your baby's body. Find other ways to have fun and other beverages to enjoy. Maybe you'll find you don't miss the alcohol anyway.

Change #5: Social Life

Having a baby brings a sudden shift in the ways you socialize (or don't). You can't go out at night, because you need to put the baby to bed. You end up staying home a lot. It's the result of being totally exhausted and completely tied down, with an entirely new routine. You also have a different mind-set: you are smitten with your new baby and don't want to leave him anyway. It's safe to say that after having one or more babies, you don't see your old social circle as much anymore, and while you may keep in touch, you may also drift apart. Instead, you tend to have playdates with other parents and their babies, although those can taper off, too, if people have trouble scheduling: everyone is so busy. That's especially true for Mom when she returns to work and has to juggle work and home life. I certainly don't see my friends like I used to, and I miss them. I do keep in touch with my closest ones, but we don't get together as often as I'd like. Life gets in the way!

Change #6: Pets

While it's fine, even great, to have pets when you have a baby, the pet may feel a little neglected as parents lavish attention on the new baby human in the house. Pet care becomes more of Daddy's job for a while.

Please never plan to get a *new* pet while you're settling in with a new baby. You just won't have the time to nurture, train, and raise two species of baby at once!

So yes, life changes, and it is sad to say good-bye to your old lifestyle. But somehow, when you're immersed in the new one, it's *not* so sad. It's actually really, really happy. With a new baby comes a new family, and a new lifestyle is born. What's important to you also shifts. Instead of late nights and dancing or movies with friends, you get picnics at the park and pajama nights with popcorn on the couch. My family and I just took up bike riding. Instead of solo gym workouts, on weekends, we're biking around (baby seats attached) as a group. It's really fun! Spending time together this way is fulfilling, special, and full of moments you'll want to treasure forever.

CHAPTER 6

The Gear

It's going to be a girl? But we paid for a boy!

—T., AGE FOUR

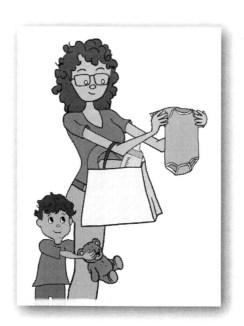

When you begin a new life together and build a home with someone you love, you need to buy furniture, dishes, linens, and so forth. When you build a new life with your baby, you need tons of gear ... again! Some items are more useful than are others—and some are essential. I'm listing them here by category; the asterisked items are personal favorites that I highly recommend, and would not do without. I've also created a list of things *not* to buy, so you can save money and limit the vast amount of stuff you need to start accumulating.

Obtaining these items will likely seem overwhelming at first, not to mention very expensive. You'll wish you had a million dollars![33] ♪. Assuming you don't: shop at secondhand and gently used clothing stores; you can find fantastic deals. Ask friends or relatives for baby items they're finished with, and be sure to register a wish list before your baby shower. (So much fun!) Yard sales and buy-and-sell websites are other good bets. Get creative in your hunting and have fun getting ready for that tiny, ridiculously costly little baby!

To Buy/Borrow/Somehow Acquire

Pregnancy

- *Essential fatty acids, fish oils (no mercury) or flax seed oil safe for pregnancy and breastfeeding
- Antacids
  - o For heartburn in third trimester
- Prenatal multivitamin with folic acid
  - o Note: It is important to start taking folic acid even before you get pregnant. I have read that fathers should also take folic acid, starting three months before conception[34]. My husband did.
- *Diclectin (prescription, Canada, available in other countries under other names), for morning sickness.
- Vitamin B_6
  - o If you do not want to take medication, or if Diclectin is not available, B_6 may also help curb nausea.[35] Be sure to take the recommended dosage. Ask your doctor or midwife.

---

33 "If I Had a Million Dollars," The Barenaked Ladies, *Gordon*, 1993, Reprise Records.

34 http://www.whattoexpect.com/preconception/ask-heidi/folic-acid-and-male-fertility.aspx

35 www.babycenter.com/404_does-vitamin-b6-help-relieve-morning-sickness_2519.bc.

- Maternity clothes
  - o It's fun to go shopping for a completely new wardrobe. Note: consignment baby/children's clothing stores usually have a maternity section with affordable pricing.
  - o Nursing bras. You will need five to six of them, but only buy one while you're pregnant; you won't know your correct size until three to four days after the birth, when your milk comes in.
  - o A few very, very long undershirts. In all four pregnancies, when I was very far along, my belly jutted out enormously; I had a little shelter that would protect a few small children from the rain if they stood underneath. The underside of my belly often felt cold, as my shirt wasn't long enough to cover it or tuck in. I found some awesome long undershirts that hugged my midsection beneath whatever top I was wearing.

Birth and Hospital Stay

Pack enough supplies for your estimated length of stay: one day or less if you have a midwife, two to three days for a conventional doctor-assisted birth, three full days for a C-section.

- *Stool softeners
- Maxi pads
  - o Super-extra-long, large.
  - o Note: cotton-topped pads are less irritating on the sensitive area with stiches than are plastic-covered pads.[36]
- *Ice pads
  - o Maxi pads that are soaked in water and frozen. Some hospitals provide them; they provide heavenly relief!
- Hemorrhoid cream
  - o If you are unfortunate enough to have the painful problem of hemorrhoids (like I did ☹), I recommend a prescription medicated foam treatment. My midwives prescribed one

---

36 Claudette Leduc, RM, and Lisa Weston, RM

when over-the-counter medicated creams and ointments weren't working. The foam was much more effective.

- Lip balm
  - o   Your lips get dry from all the heavy breathing.
- Slippers
- Pajamas
- *Cleansing bottle (provided by hospital)
  - o   For cleansing vagina and anus after using the washroom (in place of wiping because it can be painful- like using a portable bidet.)
- Sitz bath tub (may be provided by hospital)
  - o   A small tub that fits in toilet boil to cleanse.
  - o   Use with Epsom salts and very warm water.
- Newborn diapers
- Olive oil
  - o   Layering the oil on Baby's bottom can make the first few sticky bowel movements (meconium) easier to remove from his skin.[37] Olive oil is gentle and nonirritating.
  - o   I used a small container with a squirt top. That way, you don't need to find room for a large bottle of olive oil on the changing table.
- Sleepers
  - o   (one piece pajamas with feet)
- Baby scratch mittens
  - o   (mittens that cover hands so Baby's finger nails cannot scratch face)
- Receiving blankets
- Onesies
- Infant hats (for warmth)
- Camera or Smartphone and charger
  - o   Make sure the memory card is empty, and the battery should be full.
- Car seat
- Pillow and blanket for partner

---

37 Claudette Leduc, RM, and Lisa Weston, RM

- Exercise ball—large
  - o I did not find it comfortable to sit on one of these dur-
    ing labor—too much pressure "down there." But another
    mom I spoke with absolutely swore by her exercise ball
    for use during labor. She sat on it during the early stages,
    leaning against the hospital bed; her midwife or husband
    sat behind and pushed her hips together during contrac-
    tions, which helped her endure the pain. She rocked back
    and forth on the ball, and her husband rubbed her back
    between contractions. You may want to consider it if you
    are planning a natural birth (with no epidural).[38]
- Snacks and drinks
  - o Husbands tend to get grumpy when hungry. Mom will
    appreciate juice boxes and Gatorade—you may not feel
    like eating during labor, but you will be very thirsty.

Breastfeeding

- *Nursing pillow, firm
  - o A regular pillow just won't do the job. Nursing pillows—
    big, fluffy, half-doughnut shaped—are perfect for holding
    and supporting your baby in just the right spot for com-
    fortable breastfeeding. One of these is a must!
  - o Comes in handy to rest behind and around Baby when she
    is learning to sit up. It cushions the fall from multiple angles.
- *Nursing shawl
  - o Much better than a blanket for concealing your breasts, it
    has a strap that goes around your neck to avoid awkward
    slippage while you are juggling your baby around on your
    jugs. ☺ A good nursing shawl is very wide for complete pri-
    vacy and lightweight enough not to make you excessively
    hot. (You'll be hot a lot with that little warm body constantly
    snuggled up against you.) A wire curves the fabric outward

---

38 Ellen Ryan-Chan, teacher and mom

above the baby's head, so you can peek at each other and Baby can get plenty of air.

- *Vitamin D drops
  - o Nursing babies must be supplemented with vitamin D[39]. Be sure to buy vitamin D drops that are concentrated and have no added dyes or flavors. My babies hated the unconcentrated kind: it contained too much liquid per serving, it dripped out of their mouths, they didn't know how to swallow it, and it tasted strongly of cough syrup— who knows what chemicals it contained. D drops provide all the vitamin needed in just one tiny unflavored drop that goes on your nipple once a day, and your baby sucks it off without even noticing it's there.
- *Lecithin capsules
  - o If you are prone to mastitis or clogged ducts, these help prevent painful breast infections by thinning out the milk and making it less sticky.[40]
- Heating pad
  - o Helps aid in pain relief when you have engorged breasts, or if you have a clogged milk duct or mastitis.
  - o My favorite heating pads are made of fabric and filled with flaxseed; they heat up quickly in the microwave and can easily mold to the shape of your breast. You can get these heating pads with straps attached. I used a scarf to tie to the straps, and in turn, tied it around my body in just the right way so the heat was applied to the tender area.
- Nursing bras
  - o Buy just one until your milk comes in and you know your true size.
- Nursing pads
  - o You can find disposable or reusable cloth. I preferred the cloth.

---

39 www.mayoclinic.org/healthy-lifestyle/infant-and-toddler-health/expert-answers/vitamin-d-for-babies/faq-20058161

40 http://www.breastfeedinginc.ca/content.php?pagename=doc-BD-M

- *Breast pump
- Breast milk storage bags
- *Deep chest freezer
  - o A big freestanding freezer, rather than top-of-fridge one.
  - o Comes in handy if you are planning to freeze and store breast milk. It's large enough to accommodate your supply, but it also gets cold enough to keep the milk for up to a year (see chapter 14).
- *Glass bottles
  - o BPA- and chemical-free are the safest for the baby.
  - o The four-ounce size is nice and small, perfect for one serving, so you don't waste milk. It's easier for the baby to hold and drink from independently than the larger bottles.
- Nipples for bottles
- Bottle brush
- Breastfeeding undershirt, Naked Nursing Tank
  - o A handy Canadian-invented undershirt that covers your tummy but leaves your breasts exposed. Wear it under your shirt so you can breastfeed while your belly and back are still covered up for privacy.

Bottle-Feeding/Formula-Feeding

- Glass bottles with valve, eight-ounce size
- Bottle brush
- Bottle drying rack
- Bottle warmer or electric water heater and warmer
- Cooler/lunch bag
- Ice packs
- Formula (if not using breast milk)
- Formula divider travel container
- Pacifier

Diapering

- Diapers
    - o Note: you can purchase all natural, unbleached disposable diapers (better for the earth and apparently gentler on skin) however these tend to be more expensive.
- Overnight diapers (twelve-hour protection)
    - o Not necessary until six to eight months because babies begin to wet more heavily as they approach this age.
- Wipes
- Cloth diapers
    - o Cloth diapers are environmentally friendly and much more cost-effective than disposable diapers. They require a bit more work but not as much as you might think. See "Diapering Baby" (chapter 19) for more information. Note: You'll still need to use a disposable diaper at night, or you'll be up all night changing diapers. Additionally, I always packed disposable diapers in the diaper bag. Who wants to carry around dirty diapers all day? (Besides, there's no extra room in the diaper bag anyway!)
    - o Biodegradable diaper liners
        - ▪ These are sold in a large roll and are flushable. Made of a thick, soft paper product, they enable you to lift out solid waste, protecting the cloth from getting too soiled. I used these after my babies started solid foods. While not foolproof—sometimes they get all bunchy or fail to catch half the poo—they can greatly help minimize scrubbing.
    - o So many nice kinds of cloth diapers are available now, with tons of different brands online.
    - o Tucking cloth diaper liners into the diaper can also add absorbency.
- Diaper pails
    - o Only if using cloth diapers.
    - o The bucket kind with a lid is what you'll need—at least three of them (sufficient room to hold soiled diapers for up to three days, at which time they'll all be washed.)

- Borax or Amaze (by Sunlight) and jugs of white vinegar
  o Use to soak cloth diapers; also good for soaking stained clothes.
- Olive oil
- Small squeeze bottle for olive oil
- Zinc oxide cream
- Change pads
- Swim diapers
  o Use these if you plan to take Baby swimming (after five months old, when she can hold up her head).
  o Disposable and reusable types; you'll find it helpful to get both. Disposable swim diapers are useful if you need to change baby to bathing suit, and then walk around on dry land prior to swimming. Use reusable swim diapers when Baby will get wet right away. Note: reusable/cloth swim diapers do *not* hold pee in—they are effective for holding poo, but pee comes right out and into the world!
- Baby powder (use cornstarch-based, not talcum powder, for health reasons[41])
- Unscented baby lotion

Furniture and Paraphernalia

- Changing table
- Changing-table mattress
  o Get one with good curvature to encourage the baby to stay put and not roll off or out—shaped like a boat, lower in the center and higher at the edges.
- Crib
- Crib mattress
  o Firm is best.
- Breathable bumper pads (Safety First)

---

41 Shalimar Santos-Comia, RN and mom

- Two playpens, with bassinet
  - One of these doubles as a bassinet to be set up in parents' room for the first four months of the baby's life. It's handy to set up another downstairs, so you have a place for Baby to nap there. A bassinet-playpen is also great to take to a hotel to be sure of safe sleeping "quarters" that are up to code.
  - You can also use the changing table attachment on your main floor in a convenient spot.
- High chair
  - Get one with these features:
    - Easy to fold and store
    - A large tray easily removed with one hand
    - A seat that can recline for little babies or be upright for bigger babies
    - A washable seat made with waterproof fabric that wipes clean (or even better, can be removed for washing)
    - A comfy seat
    - Does not have a space between seat and stand where chubby little arms can get stuck (mine has this, and it has literally been a pain)
- Two bouncy chairs
  - Put one in the bathroom to keep Baby occupied and happy while you shower and one in the kitchen for while you are cooking.
  - Age zero to five months.
- *Two ExerSaucers
  - Same as above—but for when Baby is older.
  - Age approximately four months to sixteen months.
- Baby swing
- Baby Jumper
  - Attaches to door frame, has large springs so Baby can use his legs by bouncing again and again and again (hilarious, and good exercise for Baby).

- Baby gym
  - Not actually, a gym per se, this is basically a mat with dangly things for the baby to gaze at and grab with his cute, chubby hands. It's only useful for a short time; once babies start crawling, they've moved on. But it's a good source of fun and visual stimulation and may help promote eye-hand coordination.
- Mobile for changing table
  - Most mobiles are made to fit on cribs—I prefer to attach mine to the changing table. That's where you really need to keep your baby occupied so she'll stay still enough for you to change her diaper!
  - I like the clip-on ones (easy to attach), with toys that are easy to grab.
- Rocking chair
  - The "glider" is a very popular rocking chair for nurseries. This chair is *OK*. I have one in my baby's room. However, the glider presents some problems. The armrests are often wood, therefore hard and uncomfortable for Mommy's arms when she is breastfeeding and holding Baby. Additionally, Baby can bump his head on the wood from time to time. The big gap between armrest and chair cushion is a spot where Baby's feet can get stuck when he grows longer. Additionally, this style of chair doesn't recline much, so if Mommy is nursing at night and nods off, the head-bobbing thing happens, which is annoying and hurts. My favorite chair for night-nursing is my grandmother's old, soft, cozy rocking chair. It's out of style and a weird shade of green, but it is so comfortable: the arms are completely filled in with cushiony softness, and it reclines just enough for me to rest my head back without it falling forward if I nod off.
  - Optimal traits for a rocking chair:
    - Soft armrests with no gaps
    - Reclines slightly
    - A foot rest (optional)

- o When you're shopping for a rocking chair, bring your nursing pillow and sit down on the chair with it in your lap. If you are getting a glider, you will want an extra-large nursing pillow, to cover the hard armrests completely.
- Airplane/travel pillow
  - o You will be spending lots of time in the rocking chair, and you may fall asleep in it from time to time. An airplane/travel pillow supports your head and prevents kinks in your neck.
- Exercise ball—large
  - o Rather than for labor (uncomfortable for me, though some like it) or for exercising (ha! who has time for that?), this big ball actually makes a very effective and flexible foot-rest to use along with your rocking chair. If you don't have a chair with a footrest, get one of these for sure!
- Baby bathtub
- Nonslip bath mat
- Protective cover for tap in bathtub
  - o Blow-up style
- Shower nozzle with hose so Mom can rinse hard-to-reach places after healing from birth
- Baby gates
  - o Essential for any area with stairs (top and bottom of stairs).
  - o One for Baby's room. When your child becomes a toddler and transitions to a big bed, he can climb out. A baby gate on the bedroom door at least keeps him in the room! Gauge your baby's personality. See chapter 35, "Transition to the Big-Kid Bed."
- *Music-playing device
  - o I always play classical music at naptime and bedtime; I find it helps the kids relax and is an auditory cue that it's time to sleep. It also drowns out other household noises that may distract them or keep them awake.
- Vaporizer or humidifier

- Mats for floor
  - o If you have a hard floor (especially if you don't have carpets), mats can make the floor more comfortable for those closest to the ground.
  - o Useful for tummy time, when baby starts to sit up (so she won't keep falling backward on the hard floor), and when baby starts to roll over and crawl.
  - o I used hard foam mats that fit together like puzzle pieces. These are very affordable and easy to find at your local department store.
- "Fencing" kit
  - o We called our version The Octagon—a connected group of baby gates that, unfolded and locked, functions like a little pen. At age ten to eleven months when Baby no longer wants to be contained in the ExerSaucer, baby jumper, or playpen, it's useful to have a place for him to hang out safely with some toys when you're busy with tasks like cooking dinner. He can even hold on to the sides and stand up, and he especially loves it when older siblings join him inside! The Octagon was highly helpful for me.
- Hamper
  - o Baby clothes are little, but babies go through so many outfits each day—spit-ups, poos—you will fill up the hamper in no time!
- Potty (portable)
- Potty seats
  - o These rest on top of regular toilet seats but make the seat smaller, so kids don't fall in.
  - o You'll need as many as you have toilets.
- Step stool(s)
  - o When your baby becomes a toddler and needs to reach the sink, toilet, and big-kid bed, the stool will help him get there.
- Bed rail
  - o The rail attaches to a big-kid bed, when your toddler transitions out of the crib.

o   The rail prevents toddler from rolling out of bed in the night.
- Baby book (scrapbook for photos, notes, and memories)

Clothing and Linens

- *Sleepers (one piece pajamas with feet)
  o   Be sure to buy infant sleepers with the buttons on the front. It is a huge pain to attempt to fasten buttons on the back of an infant. Newborns are too floppy to sit up straight for you to do it, and fastening buttons or snaps with one hand is tricky.
- *Onesies
  o   These nifty little undershirts have fabric that goes over the diaper. It provides an extra layer of warmth for baby and fastens with snaps.
- Baby socks
  o   Be sure to get socks with treads on the soles for ages eight months and older.
  o   Regular socks are slippery for walking.
- Mittens (no-scratch)
  o   These are important for the first month or so in your baby's life because babies scratch their little faces with their fingernails, and they don't know who's doing it! As they grow, I always take off the mittens because babies like to explore their hands and suck on their fingers. My daughter, Evelyn, was especially inclined to scratch her face, so I had to keep the mittens on when she was sleeping longer than I did with the boys. You'll be the judge as to when your baby is ready to go bare-handed.
- Baby hats
- Baby snowsuit
  o   Get one with built-in feet. Baby boots are impossible to find.

- o Choose a one-piece, not a snowsuit with separate pants and jacket. Putting on two puffy pieces of outerwear is a lot of needless extra wrestling.
- Crib sheets
- Crib mattress cover—waterproof
  - o Get two so you have one to use when one is in the laundry.
- Sleep bags or sleep sacks
  - o These are wearable blankets that keep your baby warm and comfortable and won't be kicked off. Additionally, since the baby wears them, they cannot accidentally cover the baby's face in the night, which you don't want to happen. Your baby needs free airflow at all times.
  - o If your baby starts to stand up and risks tripping on the sleep sack and hitting his head, get sleep sacks with built-in legs.[42] Try a Halo Sleep Sack Early Walker or sew your own.
- Knitted blankets
  - o For extra warmth I always used knitted blankets, since the holes provide ventilation for breathing in case they accidentally end up on Baby's face.
- Fitted playpen sheets
- Fitted changing table sheets
- Receiving blankets—several
  - o These are multipurpose thin blankets. I always had at least three—one in the diaper bag. They have many uses: a burp cloth, to cover Baby in a car seat and stroller, to lay Baby down on, for an extra-cozy layer when you're holding a newborn, to keep them really warm and snuggly…you'll need them!
- Baby towels with hood
- Baby washcloths
  - o You will need many of these.

---

42 Tamara Adamson, teacher and mom

- Bibs
  - o You'll want two different types: small, soft ones for drool and large, plastic ones for feeding. (When you get to solid foods, it's messy.) I found a variety of bibs that fasten on the side at the baby's neck. These are awesome, being much easier to fasten than the traditional ones that fasten at the back. Snaps or dome fasteners are best; Velcro can lose adhesiveness after many washings and come undone, irritating Baby's skin. Forget bibs that tie—those should be outlawed!
- Sun hats
- Leather slippers
  - o These are great to prevent slipping with socks. They're easy to put on and take off, and they don't fall off.
- Cute baby clothing
  - o Note: At least for my babies, infant clothing sizes are way off. My babies were always a few months ahead of the sizes. Hello, chubby babies! They were wearing three-month clothes at one month, six-month clothes at three months, etc.
  - o I always shop for kids' clothes at consignment or second-hand stores. The prices are outstanding, and you'll find good-quality clothing.
  - o Chose clothing without tags, as tags can be very irritating to babies and young children.

Baby on the Go

- * Wrap-style infant carrier
  - o This style of infant carrier is far more comfortable than are the expensive name-brand infant carriers with hard straps all over the place. With the wrap, the weight of the baby is dispersed evenly throughout the stretchy fabric, making it very comfortable for Mom and Baby and easy on Mom's back. It seems complicated to fold and put on at first, but you quickly

learn how to do so. This is the best carrier! It's good for walks, day trips, the mall, or at home. Your hands are free, and the baby is safely snuggled on your chest. You can position your baby facing you when she is really little (under two months old) or sleepy. You can position her facing out so she can see the world when she's older and wants to see what's going on.

- o   In the winter, I'd put my baby in the wrap-style carrier and then put my big, fluffy maternity jacket over us both. Just his/her little head would be sticking out. It was a great way to ensure my baby was warm when we were out in the cold. My body heat kept the baby super cozy.

- *Baby sling
  - o   *A fitted, snug baby sling is very handy, comfortable, and stylish. It's good for stepping out, shopping, visiting, or using just around the house, particularly in the infant stage. The baby can easily be put in and taken out, yet is held securely so you have one hand free to deal with other kids, make sandwiches, and the like.
  - o   A large, adjustable side baby sling is helpful for larger babies and those over ten months old. It holds the child firmly on your hip, freeing you up a little to shop or hold an older sibling's hand. It's also adjustable to the size of your baby or toddler and can fit over a winter jacket.

- *UV mesh stroller cover
  - o   Sunscreen isn't recommended for babies under six months old, so this item is very useful in the summer.
  - o   The cover also doubles as a bug net.

- *Warm snuggly bag for stroller or sled
  - o   Like a sleeping bag that fits into the rider compartment, this is an awesome layer to keep Baby warm during outdoor winter activities.

- Stroller
  - o   Notes for picking a useful stroller:
    - ▪   Consider whether you want more children in the near future; if so, get a stroller that can morph into a double via an attachment. Or get a double stroller right from

the start. Otherwise, you'll end up buying a completely new double stroller in a few years and donating your beautiful single model to charity—that's what we did.

- It should have a large, accessible basket underneath. You will be stuffing in lunch bags, water bottles, towels, bathing suits, toys, extra clothes, diapers, jackets—you get the idea! My stroller has a big basket, but it's very difficult to get to; learn from my mistake.
- Big wheels. Large wheels are extremely helpful in the winter (we *can* go over that snow bank!) and for smooth riding in general.
- Make sure the seat reclines nicely so Baby can sit up or lie down easily and without too much fiddling around on your part.
- A large sunshade is very useful. The sun shining in Baby's eyes makes him cry.
- Check out the additional features: cup holders, rain covers, ride-along attachment (for little children to stand on), or the ability to double as a bassinet or laundry bag (wow!).
- You need a stroller that can carry an attached infant bucket-style car seat. When Baby is little, you can bring him around everywhere without disturbing his precious sleep.
- Test if you can push it with one hand; you'll be pushing the stroller with one hand and holding your toddler's hand with the other.
- See how easy it is to fold up and how heavy it is to lift. I absolutely love my huge, big-wheeled, luxury double stroller. (I can fit all four kids in there, if they squish.) But I have to be honest, it's a b&#$! to lift into the back of my van!
- Check to see if it fits through a standard-size door. (The door to the store you are in will work.)
- Consider its resale value. Your stroller is a big purchase; it would be nice if you can recoup some of the cost in a few years.

- Clip/hook to fasten shopping bags to the stroller handlebar or attach extra bags for day trips. (You will soon learn how to travel with *lots* of stuff.)
- Infant car seats
  - Bucket-style for children up to eight months old
    - Clicks into stroller nicely to allow Baby to sleep and stay asleep when you're out and about.
  - Three-in-one baby car seat, from eight or nine months to one year.
    - Rear-facing until baby is about twelve months old and can walk on his own.
  - Booster car seat, for ages four to nine.
    - You can postpone this one until your child is four or five years old.
- Pool noodle
  - May be needed for correct positioning of bucket-style infant seat. Check with local police/fire/community center for more information.
- Car window shades
  - These can suction cup to the windows, or perhaps your car comes with them already installed—essential to keep sun out of Baby's eyes.
- Booster high chair seat with tray (not the same thing as the booster car seat noted above)
  - For restaurants or friends' houses (keep it in the car).
  - Or you can use a funky fabric infant chair that unfolds onto a regular chair.[43] I never had one, but my friend Tamara did, and it's awesome! You don't have to lug the bulky booster seat around; just fold this fabric chair, keep it in your diaper bag, and you're good to go. The only drawback is that it doesn't have a tray, and since the baby is too short to reach the table, you'll either have to delay or stop eating to feed him or pass him little pieces of food throughout the meal.

43 Tamara Adamson, teacher and mom

- *Baby place mat with suction cups
    - o Sticks to the table to use instead of a plate (baby will drop and/or throw plate on floor and break it). Use at restaurants to guarantee a clean eating surface and for when Baby is big enough to sit in restaurant high chairs (which rarely have trays) without falling out.
    - o This mat can be useful at home, if baby rejects the high chair and wants to sit in a booster seat at the regular table like everyone else, but still has issues with throwing plates!
- Diaper bag
    - o Get one that has these features:
        - Is LARGE
        - Opens and closes easily with one hand
        - Has lots of pockets
        - Has bottle holders on the sides large enough to fit Mom's water bottle
        - Has a separate removable changing pad and a large external pocket that the pad fits into
        - Has a large, comfortable strap for your shoulder
        - Has large, zippered pockets on the outside for quick-grab items such as a nursing shawl and baby sling
        - Consider a back-pack style diaper bag, as this allows hands to be free, which is extremely helpful
    - o What to pack in the diaper bag:
        - Diapers
        - Two or three extra outfits
        - Two bibs
        - wipes
        - Zinc oxide cream (travel size)
        - Tissues
        - A few small toys
        - Hand sanitizer
        - Plastic bags (for dirty clothes and dirty diapers—avoid leaving stink bombs in others' garbage cans)
        - Sunscreen (see note below)
        - Lip balm with sunscreen

- Saline solution eye drops (these have been helpful many times—for sand in the eye, chlorine irritation, soap, etc.)
- Bandages
- Receiving blankets
- Nursing shawl (a cardigan worn backward can stand in)
- Baby sling
- Water bottle for Mom (your body is now a milk factory and the main ingredient is water; you'll be very thirsty)

Caring for Baby

- *Ear thermometer
  - Digital, fast, and easy to use
- Pedialyte liquid and a frozen ice pop mold (for when baby is older—toddler age)
- Baby fever/pain medication
  - I like the dye-free variety that lasts for up to eight hours
- Saline solution nasal spray
- Saline solution eye drops
- Baby nail clippers
- Baby bath liquid—no tears
- Baby sunscreen—no tears
  - Select a sunscreen that's all natural (if possible).
  - Babies under six months old should not wear sunscreen.
- Olive oil
  - Good for treating cradle cap
  - Useful for diapering; however, it's a bit drippy.
- Infant finger toothbrush
  - Put a single chopstick in your toothbrush holder and place the finger toothbrush on it. This is a nice way to store the finger toothbrush with the other family toothbrushes.
- Infant toothpaste (fluoride-free—use until your child turns three and can spit effectively)

- Teethers (three)
  - o Sophie the Giraffe is a famous, nontoxic teether.
  - o Get the ring kind filled with water that you can put in the fridge.
- Tiny baby hair elastics
  - o If you have a girl
- Baby powder (cornstarch, not talcum based)
- Zinc oxide cream
  - o For bad diaper rashes, extra strength with 40 percent zinc is the most effective.

Feeding Solid Foods

- Stainless-steel sippy cups
  - o Small cups are easy for Baby to hold.
  - o BPA- and chemical-free are safest.
  - o Insulated sippy cups will keep milk cold.
  - o Get two—one for milk and one for water.
- Bottle straps, two
  - o These are handy—put the bottle or sippy cup in them and attach to high chair or stroller so Baby can't throw it on the floor.
- Baby spoons
- Baby bowls
- Travel bowls
- Snack container with opening so older kids can help themselves without spilling
- Blender
  - o For making your own baby food
- Organic jarred baby food
  - o Healthy and easier than making your own!
- Ice cube trays
  - o Use for freezing your homemade baby food in one-serving portions.
- Bibs

- Washcloths
- * Rice husks for snacking
- *Nutrios (dry cereal with extra vitamins)
- Whole-grain or flax waffles
- SunButter
  - o   A yummy alternative to peanut butter

What NOT to Buy

- Pacifiers
  - o   Note: If you are breastfeeding on demand, there is no need for a pacifier. *But,* if you are bottle-feeding; your baby will likely need a pacifier.
- Crib bumper pads (traditional)
  - o   Traditional bumper pads (thick, unporous pads) can be a risk factor for SIDS, as they prevent proper airflow into the crib. (SIDS stands for sudden infant death syndrome; where babies have died unexpectedly while sleeping).
- Quilts, nonbreathable blankets
  - o   These also inhibit airflow.
- Strappy, name-brand infant carriers
  - o   These are uncomfortable and hurt your shoulders.
- Diaper pail for disposable diapers
  - o   These always get so disgustingly stinky! They have fancy gadgets that keep them closed, but when you catch a whiff as you briefly open it to put the soiled diaper in, the rotten stench will all but knock you over. I disposed of my fancy pail right along with the dirty diapers. I found it much better just to use a plastic bag hanging on the inside of the bathroom doorknob or a regular garbage can in the bathroom. If you have a toddler and are concerned about your toddler playing with a plastic bag on the doorknob, then hang it on top of the door, with an over-the-door towel hook. Each night, or whenever a stinky poop went in, I'd just tie up the bag and toss it in

the garbage in the garage. This practice eliminated terrible stenches from my house.

- o Plastic bags are much more affordable!
- Infant pants (if your baby is chubby, like mine)
  - o My babies were all so chubby that pants with a waistband were too tight and squished their soft little tummies—that couldn't feel good! I always dressed my infants in sleepers, overalls, and one-piece jumper-type outfits (these are so cute!), which don't put pressure on Baby's soft, pudgy middle.
  - o When babies grow, they stretch out, getting proportionally slimmer around the waistline. My babies were ready for pants around the ten- to twelve-month mark.
- Infant outfits with buttons or zippers down the back
  - o It is very difficult to zip or button when a floppy baby can't hold up her own head.
- Infant outfits or tops with hoods
  - o Hoods get in the way when Baby is lying down to sleep (and Baby will be lying down most of the time). Besides being lumpy for sleeping, a hood can also be dangerous: if it gets stuck on Baby's face, it could obstruct breathing. For tiny infants, I avoid anything that could cover her face. I wound up taking scissors to the cute hoodies I had.
- Baby turtlenecks
  - o Little necks already have enough folds of chubby skin, so there is no room for excess folds of fabric.
- Infant two-piece snowsuit
  - o Get the one-piece instead; it's much easier!
- Infant shoes (before five months)
  - o All I dressed my tiny infants in were sleepers—pajamas with feet. Shoes won't fit over them. When my babies got big enough for real clothes (five months), then I bought shoes.
- Nose suction bulb
  - o Not very effective.
  - o Use the method I describe in chapter 23, "Fussy Baby" (Boogers section), to clear Baby's nose if you want results!

- Mobile for the crib
  - o Babies are always sleeping in the crib, so they won't even see a mobile if you put it up. A mobile will come in handier for distracting baby over the changing table.
- Plastic bottles
  - o You don't want to warm up anything in plastic—even if it's BPA-free, you don't know what chemicals are leaching into the baby's milk.
- Eight-ounce bottles
  - o I found these were too big; I preferred the smaller four-ounce bottles. Because my babies were exclusively breastfed, the smaller bottles were enough for one serving of milk when they eventually did drink from a bottle. A smaller serving is fresher and easier to hold and drink.
- Manual breast pump
  - o Difficult to use.
- Hair barrettes (for girls)
  - o My daughter and other toddler girls all seem to dislike and pull these out, or the barrettes fell out of their fine baby hair. Go with tiny elastic bands; they stay in much better.
- Toys/stuffed animals
  - o Do not bother buying any of these ahead of time; you will accumulate so many toys quickly. Birthday gifts will set you up with more toys than you know what to do with… and just wait until Santa starts visiting!

That's it for gear! Get shopping. Remember—you don't need *everything* all at once. You can acquire the toddler items later. You may need to pace yourself!

CHAPTER 7

Doctor or Midwife?

> Don't look at my privacy.
> —E., AGE TWO

O ne of the first decisions you will make as a parent-to-be is whether to use a doctor or a midwife for your prenatal care and delivery. In some places, you are free to use both; in others, like Canada, you may only be allowed to choose one.[44] Doctors and midwives are both licensed to care for pregnant women and deliver babies. Both can see you for routine prenatal appointments; order ultrasounds, genetic screening, and blood and urine tests to monitor the growing baby's progress; and prescribe medication. The decision really boils down to which approach best fits with your personality and what priorities matter most for your birth plan. I have used both types of providers and can shed some light on what to expect. Here are some variables that can help you make the most informed choice, one that is right for you and your baby.

Midwives

Midwives are nurturing caregivers who see you for a longer time span than a doctor normally does. They will care for you all throughout

---

44 http://www.whattoexpect.com/blogs/motherhoodloomswheresmyyarn/midwife-vs-obgyn-it-doesnt-have-to-be-a-competition

the pregnancy, during the birth, and for six weeks postpartum. You will probably develop a long-lasting personal connection. In Canada, where I live, expectant mothers are assigned two midwives: a primary and a secondary. You will have appointments with both at different times, and both will be with you during Baby's birth.

Midwives have fewer clients at a time than doctors do, so they have more time for you and are available by phone to address questions or concerns. One of your midwives will always be on call, reachable by phone or pager.

I remember calling my midwives several times, asking, "I haven't felt the baby move in a while; should I be concerned?" or, "My baby's belly button scab is bleeding; what should I do?" A midwife responded to my call within minutes. Both were patient and caring, thoughtfully and thoroughly answering my questions and offering guidance. During appointments, midwives take their time with you, and appointments never feel rushed.

During the birth, *your* midwives (not the ones on call) stay with you the entire time and help you deliver your baby. Midwives coach you and lend emotional support; they give breathing tips, hold your hand, and motivate you; they're with you every step of the way. For the labor itself, you, the mother, have a lot of say in how you want it to happen, including whether you are lying down, squatting, or kneeling. (I did my first and most of my fourth baby's delivery kneeling, which for me was absolutely the least painful way, as there was no pressure on my back. I did not enjoy moving out of that position!) You have the freedom to move and walk around as you like—whatever helps you feel most comfortable and least in pain. You can have snacks and eat if you feel hungry. (My midwife made me toast with honey, and then when I threw it up later, she cleaned it up.) You do have the option of pain medication during contractions, although moms using midwives tend to avoid drugs in favor of less invasive methods like soaking in a warm bath. (I *loved* this.) Your own midwives, whom by now you have grown to love and trust, are there for you during this emotional, crazy moment. It is reassuring to have a familiar, friendly face see you through this intense time.

With midwifery, you also can choose whether to have your baby at home or in the hospital, or you can have both—do your early labor at home and transfer to the hospital for later labor and delivery. If you go for a hospital birth with a midwife, you again have a choice: you may go home shortly after the baby is born, or stay overnight and leave in one to three days, depending on how you and the baby progress.

Midwives help and guide with breastfeeding and postnatal care. They will teach you how to do whatever you don't know how to do with your brand-new infant (bathing, swaddling, cleaning the belly button, burping, holding, etc.) They are patient, nurturing, and ready to help.

After the baby is born, midwives make house visits for the first two weeks. They can weigh your baby at your home (with a nifty, adorable, sling-like contraption; you'll want photos), remove stiches and staples, check for jaundice, and do the baby hearing test, baby heel-prick blood test, and more. Midwives perform all the routine examinations that are required for a new baby. Having them visit you at home during this tender time is convenient. It's actually more than convenient—it's a huge relief. As a brand-new mom, with a new baby, you will not feel up to packing up tiny Baby in the car and waiting in the doctor's office, and your sore body will not be up for traveling much at first. From two weeks to six weeks after the birth, you bring the baby to the midwifery clinic for checkups. At six weeks they discharge you, and you transfer care to your family doctor or pediatrician.

Midwives are highly trained to assist in vaginal delivery with no complications—the most typical scenario. But in cases where an emergency or something unusual arises (true in three of my births, though I believe that high of an incidence is rare) you're transferred to the care of a doctor immediately. If you're already at the hospital, that just means buzzing the doctor on call; at home, you'd need a fast ambulance ride to the hospital. After the doctor delivers the baby, the midwives can often take over care again.

Doctors

It may appear that—when push comes to shove (or maybe just more pushes)—I prefer midwifery care. Truth be told, I had fantastic experiences with midwifery and an excellent experience with my doctors as well. While my providers were midwives for all four of my births (well, three and a half—more about that later), doctors ended up delivering three out of four of my babies.

Obstetrician/gynecologists are equipped and trained to handle the special situations that may come up—VBAC (vaginal birth after cesarean), emergency C-sections, vacuum births (all happened to me), and more.

While he wasn't available by phone for smaller concerns, my ob-gyn took his time with me, and appointments never felt rushed. I'm sure if I'd had a major question, I could have gotten him on the line. He explained everything clearly, joked around, and made me feel that I was safe and secure and that my baby and I were in good hands.

My doctor was not on call the day I went into labor with my daughter, but he did check in with me once during labor and once the next day after my baby was born. The obstetrician on call and two student doctors did the delivery. It was a little awkward at first—three men I did not know all gathered around my open vagina, my legs spread (one of them got squirted in the face with amniotic fluid—true story). Despite my initial embarrassment, I felt respected and cared for.

During labor, actually, you stop caring about who sees you naked—you're in a different zone and just want to get that baby out. The doctors checked in periodically, assessed my cervix, and went on to the next patient. I saw more of the nurses, who helped me with breathing and pain management. They were phenomenal—caring, helpful, and motivated—but they were a blur, and after their shifts were over, I never saw them again. I hope they know how much I appreciated them!

With a doctor as your chosen caregiver, hospital birth is mandatory, as is remaining there as an inpatient for two to three days; you're only discharged after the doctor gives the OK. The nurses on call are the ones checking you and your baby regularly for bleeding, breastfeeding progress and pain assessment, and teaching you how to bathe and swaddle your baby. Once you're home, care is up to your family doctor or pediatrician. You will need to travel to appointments, including the one routine follow-up with the ob-gyn at around the six-week mark, when you will have any remaining stiches removed and your condition assessed.

The decision of midwife versus doctor is a big one; there are important benefits to both. Midwives are long-term nurturers; doctors have the expertise for emergencies. Doctors are trained to handle high-risk situations, and I was grateful for that when I needed those skills the most. Midwives, on the other hand, are a wonderful option for personal, individualized pre- and postnatal care. This is a decision only you can make, with input from your partner/husband and family. Here's a table that lays out each option's pros and cons.

SIMILARITIES	
DOCTOR (Obstetrician/ Gynecologist)	**MIDWIFE**
• Both highly trained medical professionals • You may choose a hospital birth • You may choose an epidural	

DIFFERENCES	
DOCTOR (Obstetrician/ Gynecologist)	**MIDWIFE**
• Highly trained for special situations and emergencies	• Highly trained for a normal, complication-free birth
• You have one doctor	• Two midwives (in Canada)
• Your doctor may or may not be in attendance at the birth	• Both of your midwives will be present at the birth
• Must have a hospital birth	• May choose a hospital or a home birth
• Hospital stay of one to three days	• Hospital stay is optional; length of stay is up to you (up to three days)
• May be hard to contact with specific questions or concerns (doctors have more clients than do midwives)	• One of your midwives is always on call and can be paged with questions or concerns
• Your regular postpartum care will be transferred from the obstetrician/gynecologist to your family doctor or pediatrician shortly after the birth	• Midwives continue your care for six weeks postpartum, then transfer care to your family doctor or pediatrician

• Checkups are at the doctor's office	• Midwives will visit you at home for the first few appointments—no need to travel right away
• More likely to use epidural/Pitocin or other medical interventions	• More likely to offer a natural birth experience with drug-free pain intervention (soaking in bath, breathing), but you may ask for (and get) an epidural
• If an emergency arises, your doctor is equipped and prepared to handle it	• In an emergency, care can be transferred to a doctor and then back to a midwife after the delivery
• Doctors generally stick with prescription medications	• In addition to or instead of drugs, midwives may suggest natural alternatives such as papaya extract or almonds for heartburn
• The nurses at the hospital help with breastfeeding; a public health nurse can visit your home if you still need help (one visit is free; after that you need a paid lactation consultant)	• Midwives help with breastfeeding and coach you on baby care
• Snacks are discouraged during labor	• Snacks are encouraged during labor (if Mom is hungry)

What Is a Doula?

A doula is a childbirth professional moms may hire to help coach them throughout the delivery. They do not deliver babies; they're there to guide the mom on breathing, discomfort, and natural ways to manage the pain. I did not hire a doula, but I can see a wonderful benefit in doing so: they will work with you whether you're using a doctor or a midwife. Statistically speaking, doulas increase positive outcomes for both babies and moms,[45] raise your odds for a drug-free birth, and leave moms most satisfied with the experience overall.[46] They've even been linked to higher Apgar scores[47] (measuring the baby's alertness, blood flow, breathing, and other traits at birth). One disadvantage: health insurance doesn't cover their costs, so they're an out-of-pocket expense.

45 http://evidencebasedbirth.com/the-evidence-for-doulas/

46 Ibid.

47 Ibid.

CHAPTER 8

Home Birth

(After dumping the entire crayon bucket
and putting it on his head) Hat.
—M., AGE ONE

W hen you choose midwifery, you have yet another decision to make: hospital or home birth—or early labor at home and then the hospital for delivery. The latter is what happened with Terrek, my firstborn. I liked doing the labor at home—I walked outside, rested in my own bed, and had snacks in my own kitchen. However, I hated being driven to the hospital! I couldn't move around, and I was in pain. I did not enjoy being in the car.

I was too nervous about contingencies to plan on a home birth. But after speaking to two terrific moms who've gone that route, my friend Abigail and my cousin Gerd, I believe it deserves consideration. Their stories inspired and amazed me, and I'm relating them here so new moms can learn more about the option. It might not be right for everyone, but if I had known all of these details about home birth before I had my babies, I might have given it more thought.

People seem to think you're crazy if you plan to deliver at home, both women confess. Rest assured, these women are *not* crazy, and each looks back on her three successful home births with no regrets. They recall positive feelings, of being relaxed and calm and, literally, at home. Neither of them would have had it any other way.

Actually, Abigail hadn't planned on birthing exclusively at home. She saw a midwife, intending to labor at home and then going to the hospital for show time. But Abigail's baby had other plans! Her labors were all incredibly fast (making her a great candidate for home delivery). By the time the midwife arrived, her cervix was already nine centimeters dilated; a car ride at that point would have just meant discomfort and stress. So because Abigail and her husband already felt completely comfortable with the midwife, they decided to try to stay home. Abigail's secondary midwife came over, they grabbed a plastic tarp for the bed and some clean towels, and out came the baby! A healthy baby girl.

Then, however, Abigail ran into trouble: she couldn't deliver the placenta. When a shot of Pitocin didn't help, an ambulance came to take her to the hospital. She was seen the second she arrived—no waiting—the placenta was delivered, and she was all taken care of by the time the rest of her entourage arrived. Despite this wrinkle, Abigail says, birthing at home for her was worth it. Comparing photos from that day confirms her recollection of the two venues "feeling" very different. Same baby, same day—but at home—soft light came in through the windows, it was warm, and everyone was relaxed and calm. Pictures at the hospital looked sterile, clinical, and included fluorescent lights.

Abigail chose home birth for her second and third babies—this time feeling mentally and physically prepared. Both deliveries went smoothly, with no emergency change of plan. Afterward, the midwives stayed around for a few hours to do routine checks on Mom and Baby, chatting with Abigail and her husband, Charles. They had breakfast in bed. It was a warm, soft way to welcome a baby into the world.

Gerd decided on a home birth after hearing about a good friend's positive home birth experience and coming across an insight in a book, *Gentle Birth Choices* by Barbara Harper, RN. She paraphrases, "You go to the hospital if you're sick. Giving birth is a natural thing; you're not sick."[48] In Harper's words, "How did childbirth evolve from

48 Barbara Harper, RN, *Gentle Birth Choices* (Rochester, Vermont: Healing Arts Press, 2005), 31.

a woman-centered, integral part of home life to a hospital-centered, physician-controlled medical event? How did a natural process come to be seen as a pathological state that required the intervention of doctors, drugs, and medical technology?"[49]

Indeed, Gerd asked herself why she would want to bring a newborn baby into an environment full of strangers' germs, bacteria, and viruses. It would feel "so much better to be at home," she decided. "That is what persuaded me; that made such sense to me. It put the whole birth thing into perspective."[50] She noted that women have given birth for thousands of years with help from any available person—family and/or friends. Sure, more babies and moms died in childbirth back in that day, but today's midwives are professional and trained, have lots of equipment, and emergency hospital care is now a standard fallback.

Any further hesitation vanished after she, her husband, and the midwives attended a prenatal class. Eyeing the materials midwives bring to the home, she thought, "Wow—they have everything they need!" She felt completely at ease. Living five minutes from the hospital also brought peace of mind.

Excited about her first birth, Gerd also felt that she didn't know what she was doing. Thinking she was in labor, she called her midwife too soon, only to learn she was having early Braxton-Hicks contractions (false contractions, where Mom's belly gets extremely tight, not painful and not labor). The midwife didn't complain; she just left and returned when labor was actually happening.

Being in her own environment, surrounded by her own pillows, duvets, and other comforts of home, was a big plus. Gerd recalls, "It was really nice for me to bury my face in our own pillow and use our own towels, knowing where those towels have been and that they haven't been on some dirty hospital floor."[51] As someone who is sensitive to smells and sounds, she found the familiarity calming. Using baths and hot showers to ease labor pain, she appreciated the privacy

49 Ibid.
50 Gerd Griffin, mom
51 Ibid.

of being at home. "My tub, my shower, when laboring, for me person-ally, that was a huge thing—my detergent, my towels, my everything. It felt so good to be there, so comfortable."[52] Because she easily gets cold, especially during bodily trauma of any kind, she liked being able to adjust the thermostat as needed. She also appreciated being able to eat if she wanted to: her labors were long, and having your own fridge to raid is a cherished luxury when you're in labor! Recalling shar-ing chocolate and stories with the midwives, she feels lucky she was able to undergo childbirth at home. Looking back, she wouldn't have changed a thing.

I asked both women, "Any drawbacks?" Abigail said no—she hon-estly couldn't think of any, hospital transfer notwithstanding. Even lack of access to an epidural was a positive in her book: Since she didn't want such medical intervention going in, she didn't mind the whole option being off the table.

Gerd didn't report any negative aspects from her own experience, with home birth but did suggest possible sticking points. It's impor-tant not to set yourself up for disappointment, she feels—to consider all possibilities and accept that sometimes during a home birth, an emergency will arise where transfer of care is mandatory, and Mom will have to go to the hospital and deliver Baby with doctors and nurses. At this point, she adds, it is no longer the mother's choice: midwives know when medical intervention is necessary, and it's important to listen to them. Remember, their job is to get a healthy baby out! She believes in approaching home birth with an open mind, and on not being so set on the textbook experience that if it doesn't work out, you feel disappointed or that you failed.

It doesn't matter where your baby is born, she emphasizes; what matters is that the baby and Mom are healthy and safe. With her third baby, Gerd faced this fact head on. The baby was not in the optimal position for delivery. The midwife explained that if she was unable to move the baby to the correct position when she broke Gerd's water manually, then transfer of care would be needed. Gerd accepted that; she just wanted the baby to be born safely and successfully. As it

---

52 Ibid.

turned out, her midwife was able to reposition the baby and deliver her at home after all.

When Gerd asked her husband, Tyler, if he could think of any negatives to their home birth experience, he said, "The husband doesn't get to sleep!" We laughed—yet noted that Tyler undoubtedly got a lot more sleep at home than he would have at the hospital. He could rest in his own bed, while my husband had to sleep in an ugly old hospital chair, sitting up with a crooked neck. Sleep and rest are usually easier in your own home.

Other considerations Gerd notes: you might want to notify in-laws, neighbors, and others that you are in labor and will notify them when the baby is born. You probably don't want a clamor of houseguests while you are in labor; it might even be good (she joked) to put a Do Not Disturb sign on the door.

Childcare is another concern: If you have other kids in the house, it's a good idea to set up a plan for a trusted adult to come pick them up. While some parents do include their kids in the birth experience, it would be pretty traumatizing, Gerd suggests (and I agree) for a child to witness Mom in such severe pain.

Some logistical preparation also makes sense. You need to have food on hand for you, your husband, and the midwives. Labor can be quick or it can be long—and midwives are humans, too. Snacks, even meals, will be handy. Or order pizza! You may also want to keep your house in a somewhat clean state in preparation for the midwives, depending on your own priorities and comfort level.

If you decide a home birth is right for you, make preparations. Your midwives can provide a list of items you'll need, including a large plastic sheet, a fitted sheet, and a top sheet. You'll want pillows and blankets, clean towels, washcloths, and receiving blankets. Launder these linens extensively in hot water, following specific instructions the midwives provide.[53] Also stockpile paper towels, garbage bags, and, of course, clean clothes for Baby and yourself.[54] After the birth, with regular washing, most of the soiled linens should be reusable, although

---

53 Abigail Roberts, mom
54 Gerd Griffin, mom

Abigail remembers one sheet that wasn't. So don't use your best new silk linens for this endeavor. Prepare sheets and towels that have perhaps lived a good life, shall we say.

Whether you choose home birth or the hospital, you'll remember this major milestone forever. As Gerd notes, home birth may not be for everyone, but it is a personal choice that others should not judge. At times, when she revealed she'd delivered at home, people did weigh in, accusing her of wanting to be a "hero" and suffering unnecessary pain. But heroism, she insists, is not at all what it's about. For her, giving birth at home was a choice of peace, love, and comfort. So don't judge, and don't let others judge you. If a hospital birth is right for you, embrace it, and if a home birth appeals, go for it! This is your life-changing moment: own it.

DECISION-MAKING TABLE: HOME BIRTH VS. HOSPITAL BIRTH

ADVANTAGES

HOME BIRTH	HOSPITAL BIRTH
• Relaxed, calm environment, familiar surroundings • Own smells and sounds • Own linens—towels, sheets that have been cleaned by you with your detergent • Easier to rest (or sleep—for husband!) • After Baby is born, it's a relaxed time of chatting, snacking with midwives • Access to own bath, own shower, and more privacy • Can control temperature (thermostat, own blankets) • Avoid uncomfortable car ride to hospital while in labor • Mom can eat if she wants to	• Medical intervention is immediately available, such as a C-section or vacuum delivery • Epidural, nitrous oxide (laughing gas), and other pain medications are easily accessible • Away from household, other children, and family members • Minimal preparation required on your part, apart from packing hospital bag

DISADVANTAGES

HOME BIRTH	HOSPITAL BIRTH
• Advance work involved: preparing food, cleaning linens, readying birth site • Some cleanup involved—laundering linens, putting supplies away (midwives do the actual cleanup from the birth) • Transfer to hospital by ambulance may be necessary if an emergency arises	• Sterile, unfamiliar environment • Foreign germs, viruses, and bacteria may be present at hospital • Hospitals can be cold • Snacking is difficult or not allowed • Uncomfortable or difficult for husband to rest and sleep

CHAPTER 9

Birth Options: C-Section vs. Vaginal, Epidural vs. No Epidural

> When we were in your tummy, we
> played with your belly button.
> —T., AGE FOUR

All four of my birth experiences were completely different. My first one went according to my plan of how I had always wanted to experience birth: totally natural. My following three all deviated from the plan. All of them were magical—no matter how many children you have, it's such a miracle. How is it possible that a tiny little human can come out of your body? It's so strange when you really think about it. Here are my stories detailing each birth scenario, with my notes about the different choices. From my varied experiences with all types of labor, I hope you derive insight on what you value in a birth plan and what you may want to avoid. Get ready to push it.[55] ♪

Birth #1: All Natural

I wanted to honor Mother Nature and my body's wisdom and strength and have my baby without drugs. I didn't want medical interventions.

---

55 "Push It," by Salt 'N Pepa, *Hot, Cool & Vicious*, 1986, Next Plateau Records/London Records.

I didn't want an epidural. I didn't like the idea of a needle going into my spine, and I was worried about side effects. Instead, I used natural pain-relief methods.

I was in the care of two wonderful midwives for the first birth. When I started getting regular contractions, I phoned them, and my primary midwife came over. I underwent the early stages of labor at home, under her care. I rested in my own bed, I walked around my backyard, and I soaked in the bathtub. I snacked on toast and honey. It was nice to be at home for this part of the labor, where it was comfortable and private. We went to the hospital after my water broke in a huge gush during a contraction in my kitchen.

During labor, I focused on yoga breathing and an internal mantra of "Let your body do its job." I relied on my body, having confidence that it knew what to do, which it did. At the hospital, I went back in the tub to soak. The warm water around my body eased the pain during contractions. I leaned on my husband and midwife, and rocked back and forth. The movement helped me get through the contractions. The contractions got a lot more painful than I had ever anticipated, but with my breathing and internal focus, I was able to handle them. (Although I did tell myself that this was the last time I would be doing this, as I couldn't possibly endure this a second time. I decided in that moment that I would therefore only have one child. Lucky for my other kids, I forgot about that decision later.)

Pushing was really hard. I didn't know that there would be such an intense pressure that would make me feel like the baby was coming out of my bottom! When I needed to push, it felt like pushing out an enormous number two. This feeling was most unpleasant, and it hurt a lot! This was when my natural pain-relief methods failed, and I wanted to throw them out the window.

The one good thing about not having an epidural was that I was able to move around. I walked around and rocked all during labor, and during the pushing phase, I could change positions. The position that worked the best for me was up on my knees, leaning over the upright head of the hospital bed. I was facing my butt to everyone (not very attractive), but, by that point, my modesty had completely vanished, and I didn't care who walked in and saw me that way. My mind was in a different place.

Because of the position I was in, the first I saw of my baby boy, Terrek, were his tiny, perfect feet wiggling below me. I got to hold my baby skin-to-skin right after the birth. I was in such a state of amazement. I was also in a state of huge relief, knowing the labor was finally over. When told I had to push again to deliver the placenta, I was like, "You have got to be kidding me!" But it was nothing, and the placenta came out easily. My perineum tore during the birth, and I required stiches. But I didn't feel a thing as my midwife stitched me up. I think I was numb down there from the pain!

The biggest surprise from a natural birth, with no epidural, was how well I felt as soon as the baby was out. I wanted to get up, walk around, and take a shower. I was energized, and I felt completely fine! Of course, my midwives made me lie down and rest.

Birth #2: C-section

I had intended to deliver my second baby the same way as the first. My second son, Patrick, had different ideas. I went into labor the same way as before—at home, with the start of regular contractions. My husband and I went to the hospital earlier than previously, as my midwives expected that this time my labor would be faster. Again, my son felt differently. (A precursor to his personality. He has his own ideas about everything!)

After fourteen hours of walking around the hospital during early labor (boring, tiring, painful, yucky), something strange happened. My labor slowed down and stopped. My midwives sent me home to rest and told me to come back the next day to be checked. We went home; I ate a huge plate of spaghetti and slept like a log. My labor still had not turned back on the next day, although I had felt a great deal of fetal movement during my time at home.

I returned to the hospital to check on Baby's progress. When my midwife checked my cervix and felt for the baby's head, it was gone. She couldn't find it. We all were confounded. Hide and seek, anyone? The baby had completely moved positions. He was no longer in the head-down, ready-to-come out position. He was lying transverse across my belly. The doctor on call at the hospital confirmed it. He said I would need a C-section right away, as the baby's position could be very dangerous for both him and me if I went back into labor.

I was very nervous about the epidural, but it wasn't that bad. The anesthesiologist numbed my back first, and my husband held my hands, looked into my eyes, and distracted me with funny stories of Terrek, who was just two at the time.

The actual C-section was fast. It was more uncomfortable than I expected because I could feel them pushing and prodding at my belly, although I didn't suffer actual pain. I felt a huge gush of liquid splash all over my abdomen—probably amniotic fluid. My midwife stayed with me and held one of my hands while my husband held the other.

The first memory I have of my second son, Patrick, was his tiny cry, and my husband saying, "He's awesome, Babe. He's awesome." The doctor noted that the cord was wrapped around the baby's arm, which was probably why he moved during labor. My midwife explained that the baby could send a signal to stop labor if he's in trouble. Nature is truly amazing.

I didn't get to have immediate skin-to-skin time with Patrick because of the surgery. If you are having a C-section birth, ask that the baby be placed atop your husband for the initial skin-to-skin time.[56] This initial contact is important for your baby, a comfort after such a dramatic change in surroundings, and essential for the colonizing of healthy bacteria on your baby's skin.[57] Patrick missed this moment initially, and I wonder if that may have contributed to the allergies and asthma he developed later as a child.[58] I started breastfeeding soon after they stitched me up. I felt some of the stitching, so they gave me an extra shot of some drug, which seems to have erased my memory, because I can't remember holding my son for the first time. I remember his cries when he came out, I

56 Mary Miller, teacher and mom

57 http://www.babycenter.com/0_how-breastfeeding-benefits-you-and-your-baby_8910.bc

58 http://www.nbci.ca/index.php?option=com_content&id=82:the-importance-of-skin-to-skin-contact-&Itemid=17

remember my husband placing the baby beside my head, and then I don't remember anything until I was in the recovery room already breastfeeding.

After the C-section, I was markedly nauseated from the anesthesia. My abdomen also hurt a lot at the site of the incision. When I had to throw up, the pain in my belly was terrible. I required antinausea and pain medications to feel better. Recovery from this C-section was much slower than from the vaginal delivery. My midsection was very sore for several weeks. I couldn't lie on my side in bed because it felt like my insides were going to fall out. I wasn't able to lift my toddler for six weeks. I sensed that was very difficult for him to understand, and for me it was sad! But eventually I healed and had my new beautiful baby, and I could lift my toddler again. The pain and discomfort was absolutely the better alternative than what could have happened. The C-section might have saved my life or that of my son. We both came out of a tricky birthing situation healthy and happy. Modern medicine is truly a wonder.

Birth #3: VBAC with Epidural

When I was pregnant with my daughter, Evelyn, I was again in the care of midwives. But since I wanted to have a vaginal birth after a C-section (VBAC), I had to have a consultation with an obstetrician/gynecologist. There are risks with a VBAC; however, there are also risks with repeated C-sections. The first doctor I saw did not advise a VBAC, due to varicose veins on my uterus and a higher than average scar location. I really wanted to try a VBAC, so I got a second opinion.

My midwives referred me to specialists at a larger urban hospital. The specialist obstetrician/gynecologists there decided I was a good candidate for a VBAC. They explained that VBACs can be a safe birth option for the right candidate and can be easier on the body in the long run than can repeated C-sections. (Note: you must wait a minimum of two years between births to have a VBAC.) During labor, doctors would be watching for stress on my uterine scar, and if trouble emerged, an emergency C-section could be performed.[59] Please note

59 Dr. Howard Berger, gynecologist

that doctors must make this decision; do not make this decision on your own. The odds are great for a healthy baby and a healthy mom after a VBAC; however, my doctor did say that, "even in a hospital setting, with appropriate team and response time, there are rare cases where bad outcomes can occur."[60]

My care was transferred from the midwives to one of the hospital's ob-gyns who specialize in high-risk births. I was seven months' pregnant by then. The care I received was again excellent, though I did have to travel quite a distance for each appointment. And while my actual doctor was not present at the birth, he checked in twice to see how things were going.

My labor began differently this time. It started with a trickle of my water breaking at six o'clock in the morning. My contractions began soon after, but they were very mild. We drove to the city and checked into the hospital. My labor was very slow to progress. The contractions were mild and far apart, and I was only dilated one centimeter. It was a quiet morning in the hospital, and we were watching reruns and going for walks in my robe and slippers. Because my water had already broken, after six hours, the doctors on call (my own doctor wasn't present) decided they needed to speed things up. Once a mother's water breaks, the baby is at an increased risk of infection, so they did not want to let the labor continue at that pace. So they induced my labor by giving me Pitocin in an IV, which got things moving.

My body reacted to this hormone right away, and my contractions got bad, fast. They became so painful and intense, so quickly, that my breathing and yoga mantras were not working for me, and I asked for an epidural. This was huge for me, as I had intended to do this naturally again. (I've never been big on medications.) Oh sweet relief! The miracle of drugs! Once the epidural kicked in, it didn't even feel like I was in labor anymore. I became completely relaxed, and all the pain went away. It was heavenly. My husband and I watched *American Idol*, I rested, and it was lovely. I could still tell when I was having a contraction because of the pressure, but I felt no pain, which was fantastic! Epidurals are like magic! I couldn't believe how effective it was, and I felt like I was crazy to have not had the epidural the first time.

---

60 Ibid.

When it was time to push, I pushed with intensity, but no pain. My daughter was born quickly and easily. True, I couldn't move around during this delivery, but I didn't care. I was so comfortable and relaxed, and I was just fine in my hospital bed. I had skin-to-skin time immediately with my daughter, and I remember it all perfectly. This was overall my most positive birth experience.

Birth #4: Vaginal Birth with Vacuum Delivery and No Epidural

This type of delivery is not a method one chooses. Doctors use a vacuum only if the baby is stuck and cannot be born without additional help. Such was the case for my fourth delivery, and it wasn't fun...but it had a happy ending!

My labor started differently again this time. My contractions were very far apart (twenty to thirty minutes) for twenty-four hours. It was a very strange pattern. I kept talking with my midwife on the phone. I didn't know whether I was in labor. Then suddenly, at two o'clock in the afternoon, my contractions were three minutes apart. I phoned my midwives again, and we headed to the hospital. By the time I was admitted, my cervix was already four centimeters dilated. I was so happy! I was optimistic that this would be a faster labor and delivery than were the others.

The contractions continued steadily, and I was able to handle them with my deep breathing and by squeezing my husband's hand. "I can do this without an epidural," I thought. (I must have been temporarily insane or had some kind of amnesia—or I just have an unjustified fear of an epidural needle going into my spine.) My labor progressed quickly and five hours later, I was ready to push. When I wanted the epidural, it was too late as I was already in the pushing stage. (The epidural must be administered before it comes to this). I didn't ask for the epidural in time. Something I regretted later.

The active labor and intense contractions were bad but manageable—painful, yes, but with my yoga breathing and my focus, I was coping. I didn't even feel the effects of the back labor...yet. When the baby's head is pointed down toward the vagina but the baby's face is pointing toward the belly instead of toward the back, it is called back labor because the baby's skull hits along your spine as the baby descends, which for the mother can be incredibly painful. I didn't actually have pain in my back, and I attribute that to the position I was in. I had not had an epidural so I could move around, and for me the most comfortable position was up on my knees on the hospital bed, leaning forward over the back of the raised bed. I had my butt to everyone again (just like during my first birth experience). I had come full circle...or should I say full moon? Gravity was working in my favor and pulling the baby down toward my front, so the pressure was not on my spine. This was one benefit to not having had the epidural.

The pushing was very difficult. The fact that my baby was in the back-labor position (a.k.a. "sunny side up"), made it more difficult for the baby to come out. His head wasn't getting past my pubic bone. My midwives had to call the doctor because my baby's heart rate was dropping, and he was stuck. I couldn't get him out. I was pushing with every last bit of my strength. I was trying so hard and was worried for his safety. I changed positions, to the traditional-lying-on-back with legs up. Nothing was happening. It was really intense. The doctor on call zoomed in and delivered my baby with a vacuum. Once she got that vacuum on his head, I pushed and she pulled, and he was out within minutes. I was so thankful that it was fast.

Once my little son Maxwell was born, I was relieved to be done with the pain, and so thankful that he was OK. My tears of joy and sense of wonder kicked in when I got to hold him. He had a weird cone shape to his head because of the vacuum, but that went away quickly. He was coughing and sputtering at first because he'd breathed in liquid, so he needed suction to clear his lungs. Maxwell was my biggest baby—eight pounds and five ounces. When I got my treasured skin-to-skin time, he still seemed so tiny and precious. I was instantly in love all over again.

Now, after four completely different birth experiences, I'm: 1) very glad to be done with labor and delivery, and 2) so thankful that I did go through labor and delivery. The painful, uncomfortable interlude happens in one day that will soon be a distant memory, and you get your babies for the rest of your life. Babies are individual miracles, and I love mine more than life itself. The feeling I have for my children is stronger than anything—words cannot even begin to describe the love I have for each of them and the joy I get from each. My love for them is stronger than the pain I felt each of those four days of labor combined. So what I'm trying to say is that yes, labor is difficult, but what you get out of it is so good. It's worth it! (And if you get the epidural, it is bearable!)

While you are making your many decisions about what kind of birth you will have and mentally preparing yourself for this magnificent experience, you will also want to prepare your bag for the hospital. With my first baby, I was—let's just say—a tad overambitious with my hospital packing. (Can you hear my husband guffaw from here?) I read every list online about what to bring. I ended up with a large suitcase and a duffel bag jam-packed, including my CD player (large boom box) with relaxing music, a rolling pin for massage, and a large piece of tranquil artwork for my focal point. I had my sister drop off five pillows at the hospital (we forgot ours). My husband ended up having to tote my luggage around (and still complains about this today). How many of these "birthing" tools did I actually use or appreciate? Well, the truth is, none! All of them were superfluous. All you need is a firm hand to hold and some liquid to drink. Leave the rest up to your body. For a list of all the actually useful items you should pack in your hospital bag, refer to chapter 6, "The Gear." As for the husband who complains about having to carry the luggage, once he sees what you have to do, he'll thank his lucky stars that all he has to do is carry the luggage. You shouldn't have to punch him in the nose for him to realize you have the harder job.

With all the many choices when it comes to childbirth (doctor or midwife? hospital or home? epidural or not? C-section or vaginal?), here—after personally going through all of it—is what I recommend: A midwife at a hospital, with a vaginal delivery if possible and an epidural. With this combination, you get nurturing, personalized care, a location equipped to handle medical emergencies, available pain interventions, and a quicker recovery that is less traumatic for your body. This is the best! And don't forget to insist on your valuable skin-to-skin time. However crazy your experience winds up being, you will soon forget the downsides and remember the warm, priceless, indescribable feeling you treasured while holding your tiny newborn baby for the first time. Today is the greatest.[61] ♪

---

61 "Today," Smashing Pumpkins, *Siamese Dream*, 1993, Virgin Records.

MAIN POINTS FROM MY BIRTH EXPERIENCES

VAGINAL BIRTH WITH NO EPIDURAL

- I could move around freely.
- I felt great after.
- My recovery was quicker than with a C-section.
- It was incredibly painful.

C-SECTION BIRTH

- It was a short, painless delivery.
- It may have saved my life and/or the life of my baby. Note: with a scheduled C-section, you can plan ahead as you will know the birth date in advance. (Mine was an emergency C-section).
- I felt terrible after (my belly was extremely sore; I felt nauseated and groggy from the anesthetic).
- My recovery time was longer.
- My belly took longer to go down.
- I couldn't lift my toddler for six weeks.

VBAC WITH EPIDURAL

- It was a painless, peaceful and relaxed delivery.
- I couldn't move around during labor.
- I couldn't move around immediately after labor.

VAGINAL BIRTH WITH VACUUM DELIVERY AND NO EPIDURAL*

- My baby came out quickly.
- I felt great after.
- I could move around during and after labor.

*NOTE – avoid this option! If you know you are having back labor (harder for baby to get out and more pain), seriously consider getting the epidural.

CHAPTER 10

Care of Your Body after Birth

Mommy, your nose is so big and pointy,
it could cut a watermelon.
—T., Age Six

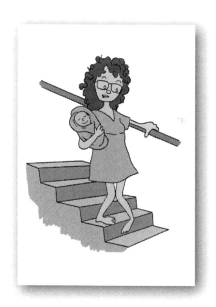

After giving birth, your body feels broken. For me, the feeling was a state of total, pure happiness, complete exhaustion, and physical pain. Your entire body hurts. Your vagina, bottom, abdomen, and breasts hurt. (It got progressively worse with each baby...poor body!) Knowing in advance can help you prepare. Your body will feel ruined but will gradually heal itself. You'll feel better after six weeks, I promise!

First, your vagina has been extremely stretched and in many cases torn or cut and has probably been stitched for repair. Taking pain medication, namely acetaminophen and ibuprofen, will help. The hospital will give you both. Alternate them so that they overlap, and you won't be without something to ease the pain at all times. When one medication wears off, the other will be just kicking in, and you won't exceed the recommended dosage for either, as you would if you only took one kind of pain medication. The best relief for your special area "down there": ice pads. Wet regular or long maxi pads with cold water and put them in the freezer. Put these on so the extreme cold will numb everything up, and it will feel heavenly. These were my number-one favorite feel-better remedy after giving birth. Prepare lots of them!

You will want to avoid rubbing with toilet paper, but of course, you want to avoid any infection, especially if you had stitches and are healing up. One solution is a hospital-provided squirt bottle for cleansing after you use the bathroom. Squirt your vaginal area with warm water after each time you use the toilet. It feels soothing and nice and relieves the pain for a few minutes, while cleaning away the germs; highly recommended.

Sitz baths are another option. Fill a small tub (specially made for this purpose) with warm water and lots of Epsom salts, place the tub on the toilet bowl, and sit in it, thereby rinsing and soaking your private areas in warm, purifying water.

It is also a good idea to air out your vaginal area after giving birth. You will be bleeding, creating a lot of moisture on the stiches. To promote healing and prevent infection, place a towel on your bed to protect the sheets and lie on it on your side, knees together.[62] Feel the breeze! This sounds embarrassing, but no one needs to know! Do it when Baby is sleeping and lock your bedroom door against surprise visitors.

---

62 Claudette Leduc, RM, and Lisa Weston, RM

You will be cautioned to avoid climbing stairs immediately after childbirth, especially if you have stiches. The movement of spreading your legs while walking up and down can tug at the stiches and prevent proper healing. I developed a stair-navigating method that looks ridiculous but didn't pull the stitches. I squeezed my knees together and stood on my toes. Twisting from my waist and keeping my crotch steady, I gently brought alternate feet down to the next step with each pivot. That way I could make my way safely around the house and didn't feel so isolated upstairs. Additionally, remember to sit with knees together. When your legs are apart, the skin around your vagina is pulled, the opposite of what needs to happen for the perineum to heal. No cross-legged sitting until everything is healed back together again!

Following a C-section, you don't have vaginal problems; instead you have a very sore section where the incision is on your lower belly. Lying on your side hurts, and it feels as if your tummy may fall out of its skin. I slept on my back at first. You won't be able to lift anything heavy for six weeks, including toddlers. Not picking up my two-year-old after I had my second son was very difficult. I had to get creative. I sat on the floor and let him climb on my lap. I had to bribe him to come up the stairs on his own after lunch for his nap by giving him his gummy vitamin once he reached the top. Then I quickly closed the baby gate behind him.

Sitting up in bed was hard. I developed a way of getting up by rolling over on my side and pushing myself up with my arms. The incision will heal pretty quickly, and after six weeks, you can get your stiches or staples removed—slightly painful but not a big deal. You need to watch your incision during the first six weeks to make sure it doesn't get red, which could indicate an infection. That happened to me, and I needed to go on antibiotics. If you have any stitches, you can't take baths or swim for six weeks, either, whether you delivered by C-section or vaginally. And be aware that a cesarean does leave a permanent scar on your lower abdomen. The scar will gradually shrink, and soon, you'll not even notice it anymore.

You will be bleeding for a while after giving birth. It's like having your period for approximately six weeks straight, so stock up with lots of pads.

A note about dissolving stitches: sometimes they *don't* dissolve. I encountered that problem. If your stitches area hurts after birth, then feels better for a while, and then begins to hurt again around the five-week mark, that may be what's going on: that the stitches are not dissolving as they should. If you feel tugging when you walk or a large knot in the threading that is irritating your skin, see your doctor or midwife and ask about having the stitches removed. For me, the process took just a few minutes and didn't hurt, although it was slightly uncomfortable, and everything felt so much better once I'd had the stitches snipped and taken out.

Many women suffer from hemorrhoids after giving birth, from the pushing or even, for some reason, following a C-section. Hemorrhoids are a huge pain in the butt...literally! Hemorrhoids are folds of the inside skin of the anus that poke out of the rectum (when really they belong inside). Short of surgical repair, they never completely go away, but they can be managed. They can be extremely painful and feel worse with each successive delivery; by my fourth baby, I was in bad shape. Again, ice pads brought the best pain relief. Over-the-counter creams didn't work for me, but a prescription medicated foam did help. Ask your doctor about a prescription hemorrhoid foam, if you too are in bad shape in this department. Some recommend an inflatable inner tube if sitting is painful, but I tried one and found it just put more pressure on the hemorrhoids by pulling my butt cheeks apart and prevented any back support by keeping me forward in the chair. It also had a terrible rubber smell.

Placing a pillow on my chair helped as long as I didn't push it all the way back in the seat, so I had a gap where my bottom could hang over, taking pressure off the sore area and letting me lean back (much needed by an exhausted new mom). The squirt bottle and sitz bath also provided much appreciated relief for the hemorrhoidal pain. Baby wipes are good, gentle (and cleansing) substitutes for toilet paper if you have hemorrhoids. Mine healed (mostly), thank goodness, two to three weeks after delivery, but they can resurface from time to time. Ice, the best remedy, is a trickier proposition at this stage, since recurring hemorrhoids aren't as large as they are right after birth; they just poke out a bit so a frozen pad may not reach. But I found a perfectly shaped ice pack for this specific purpose: freeze pops "Freezies" (small). These fit discreetly right in there where the pain is. Wrap them in a paper towel before putting them in place, and be sure to discard them after use.

When beginning to breastfeed, many women get uterine contractions. I didn't with my first three babies, but with my fourth, these post-delivery contractions were severe! Ouch. I just breathed through them. One consolation for the discomfort is knowing that they're actually working to bring your tummy in—your uterus is shrinking back to its regular size.

Your breasts won't hurt right after the birth, but they will two to four days later when your milk comes in. Get ready for some huge boobs, which unfortunately will be hard as rocks and sore at first. Pumping your breast milk can help relieve some, but not all, of the pressure. I was advised not to pump at first for fear that it would only encourage my body to continue producing this stupendous amount of milk. That was bad advice. Go ahead and pump! I didn't with my first two babies and had to endure a lot of pain in my swollen breasts.

For my second two, I went ahead and pumped, and was so glad I did. It didn't take the fullness and pain completely away, but it reduced pressure, making me feel so much better. It did not cause a problem, either; I had a lot of extra milk to freeze at the beginning, but my breasts calmed down in a few days to a week.

Heating pads and warm compresses also help. Swollen breasts are quite uncomfortable until your body figures out how much milk the baby is using and how much it needs to make. At first, your body is overdoing it, and your breasts are quite engorged. Placing cabbage leaves in your bra may be an old wives' remedy, but it's apparently also effective. When you take them out, the cabbage leaves are hot and wilted, as if they've been steamed in a pot for dinner! Your breasts will feel better in a few more days.

Massage your breasts in the shower regularly to keep the milk ducts open and the milk moving. It is common to get hard lumps during breastfeeding; breast milk can be quite sticky and get gummed up, leading to blocked ducts or even mastitis (a breast infection). Keep nursing! It's the best thing to do in order to move the milk. For more information on how to treat and care for clogged ducts and mastitis, see chapter 13, "Breastfeeding."

One odd postpartum symptom I hadn't expected was hair loss. Some of your hair will fall out (not all), but it's temporary and will not lead to baldness, so don't despair. The biggest problem is that it can clog your shower drain. Tip: Did you know wet hair sticks well to tile shower walls? Run your hands over your hair as you wring it out after shampooing and pull out the loose hair. Put it on the wall, and it will stay there. Then collect it and toss it in the garbage so your drains don't clog. You'll also frequently find strands of your hair clenched in your baby's tiny fists. No need to freak out! The hair loss will only last about four months, and no one will notice it but you.

Another possible postpartum problem is incontinence (leaky bladder).[63] Several new mothers I spoke with report having to run to the bathroom suddenly. Practicing Kegel exercises to strengthen the muscles down there can help, but to resolve fully this embarrassing and inconvenient condition, see a physical therapist (physiotherapist in Canada) who specializes in women's postnatal care for the pelvic floor.[64] Who knew such a colorful variety of Kegel exercises existed? Note: Even if you don't have bladder symptoms, pelvic floor therapy can help new moms prevent problems from developing later on.[65] In extreme incontinence cases, surgery may be needed, but try therapy first.

Leaky bladders are one thing, but a uterine prolapse is another. No joke—my old pet rat, Zinnea, had a uterine prolapse. This big bubble thing fell out of her. It was very sad, and very strange, and it did not look pleasant. According to two different US studies, uterine prolapse occurred in 11 to 14 percent of women[66]. Don't let that happen to you! Exercise all those muscles deep inside you with an assortment of Kegel exercises only a physical therapist specializing in pelvic care can teach you. The Kegels can be tricky at first, but

---

63 Nadia Ramprasad, MPT

64 Ibid.

65 Ibid.

66 http://www.ncbi.nlm.nih.gov/pmc/articles/PMC2034734/

you'll get the hang of it and will find muscles you didn't even know you had. Some of these exercises reportedly help improve the quality of your sex life as well.[67] Hmm, that's worth the extra effort right there!

Postnatal physical therapy can also improve general muscle strength.[68] After four pregnancies, my stomach muscles had literally separated and stretched out. My abdomen was like an unbuttoned sweater; it had a two-inch vertical gap where there were absolutely no muscles. A specially designed program can work these muscles so they'll go back together or at least shrink the gap.[69] My rehab program involved specific exercises, core strengthening, and wearing an abdominal binder, a device that resembles a girdle, for a while.[70]

I was also extremely sweaty for a little while after giving birth. Blame it on those raging hormones again—my entire body was dripping wet. I woke at night to feed the baby and had to change my shirt because it was soaked in sweat. My postpartum body was emitting lots of fluids—blood, sweat, tears, and milk. No wonder I was so thirsty all the time!

Emotions can be challenging in this period, too. Postpartum depression is the most severe instance, but mild cases of the weepies can occur as well. Your hormones are going crazy. You're completely exhausted from the trauma of birth and the lack of sleep from caring for your baby, and you may find it all overwhelming, crying for no apparent reason. Crying is OK! Feel free to let it all out. Make sure you communicate with friends and family and your spouse or partner. If you are feeling very sad, angry, or just not yourself, and the feeling persists, you may in fact have postpartum depression; see your doctor or midwife. Help now available for this condition includes cognitive therapy, medication, and support groups.[71] Please do reach out if you

---

67 Nadia Ramprasad, MPT

68 Ibid.

69 Ibid.

70 Nadia Ramprasad, MPT.

71 http://www.cmha.ca/mental_health/postpartum-depression/#.VXGrpFVVhHw

think you are depressed. Remember: this, too, will pass. Keep going and carry on![72] ♪

Your husband will be wondering when you will be well enough to engage in the lovely act that got you in this situation in the first place. He may ask, "When can we have sex again?" After having a baby, you won't want anything to do with sex. The thought of my husband coming near me with his penis made me close my legs together and cringe. Everything feels so damaged down there that this just does not seem pleasant or in any way humane!

Magically, your vagina does heal. Slowly—but surely—your body repairs itself and the stiches dissolve. Your hormones kick back in, and—believe it or not—by six weeks postpartum you can resume your physical relationship with your husband. He will jump for joy and do a happy dance. For you, however, it may take several times before it feels "all better" during sex. For some lucky women, sex isn't painful at all after giving birth; however, most will feel sore and very sensitive at first, especially if there were stitches. If sex is still painful after one month, then something could be up, and you might want to see the doctor.

After my first birth, my stitches area did not heal normally. There was a weird bit of skin sticking out somewhere that did not belong, which made sex continually painful. My gynecologist had to burn the skin off (a simple day procedure). After that, sex proceeded to improve dramatically! I know other women whose stitches made the vagina too tight, and it took a while to stretch back out to normal, so sex hurt for a while. Advice: use lots of lubrication, and engage in lots of foreplay! Let's get it on...[73] ♪

Additionally, the more you do *it*, the better *it* will begin to feel. It feels good to renew the connection between you and your partner. This is great not only physically but emotionally, too. Be forewarned, though, that with breastfeeding, the hormones keep your sex drive lower than usual. (Your body is saying, "What? Are you crazy? Why in the world would you do something that could get you pregnant? You

---

72 "Carry On," Fun., *One Night*, 2012, Ramen/Atlantic/Electra.
73 "Let's Get It On," Marvin Gaye, *Let's Get It On*, 1973, Tamla Records.

just had a baby!") To top it off, you are, of course, exhausted, so when you do get in bed, you desperately want to sleep, and that's pretty much all you'll want to do in bed for a while. When you muster up the energy and find the time and opportunity (all kids sleeping), watch out for leaky breasts—they don't differentiate between your husband and your baby! Your body interprets nipple stimulation of any kind as your baby sucking and will automatically produce milk. You may be the one squirting your husband before he squirts you! Ha!

One simple but vital tip for postbaby well-being: correct your posture. It is so easy to slouch forward all the time because of your extra weight in front (enlarged breasts, expanded tummy). Remind yourself to pull your shoulders back and down and to straighten your back when you are sitting and standing. You will feel and look better.

The biggest difficulty to deal with after giving birth is sheer exhaustion. Not only has your body been through a traumatic and draining ordeal, but also, you now have to wake up every two to three hours to feed and tend to the baby. Your body isn't getting the rest it needs to heal. Yet somehow, we all get through it, and you will, too. The key is resting and napping during the day. Everyone will tell you to "sleep when your baby sleeps!" That is valuable advice, but if you have other children at home, it's not always practical. This is when the TV may become handy, so you can snooze on the couch while your preschooler watches Elmo. Believe me, you'll need to find a way to squeeze in at least one nap a day. It will make a vital difference.

Your body will heal, and you *will* feel better. No, your body will never be the same as it was prebirth. You'll have scars and stretch marks here and there, but you will also have your baby: a little person you grew and made. Nature is a miracle worker. Truly.

CHAPTER 11

Hospital Stay

You're insane, like a duck.
—P., AGE FIVE

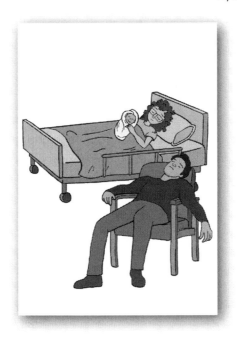

The length of your hospital stay will depend on a few factors. If you have a midwife and a normal, complication-free birth, then you don't have to stay at the hospital at all, unless you want to. However, since you will be exhausted and sore, you may not exactly be eager to jump up, get dressed, and run out to the car. I always stayed a minimum of one night at the hospital for each birth. I enjoyed that time to rest and connect with my new baby and my husband. I knew once I went home, we would be busy. It is easier to have concentrated, undisturbed rest at the hospital when you have other kids at home.

If a doctor is your care provider, you'll be required to remain in the hospital at least twenty-four hours. If you have a C-section, you'll likely stay three days.

If at all possible, see that your husband or partner can be with you for the duration of your hospital stay. You will really need him. Unfortunately, his sleeping arrangements may be pretty shabby. Picture a hard, fold-out chair with no pillow and only a thin sheet for a blanket, and then picture it awkward, flat, and skinny. You may want to bring bedding from home so he will sleep a little better.

While you are at the hospital, a nurse will monitor you and your baby. She will check your temperature, pain level, bleeding amount, breastfeeding progress, and your ability to pee and have a bowel movement after the birth. She will weigh Baby, check for jaundice, and give him a bath; conduct hearing and blood tests, and give him an injection of vitamin K. Nurses are available if you have questions or concerns. Most of them are wonderfully approachable, helpful, and kind.

Note: sometimes the nurse will want to whisk the baby away for a particular process and bring her right back. I did not feel comfortable letting a stranger whisk my baby away, even though she was a nurse and my baby wore an ID bracelet, and I insisted my husband go along whenever the baby was taken from the room. This was just a safeguard I felt I needed. I was not well enough to get up and walk in order to keep up with the busy nurse, who had lots to do on her shift. That was the perfect job for Daddy.

Additionally, keep in mind that you and your husband/partner are in charge of this baby, not the nurses. This baby is yours, and you are the boss. Don't be afraid to say no. After the birth of my daughter, I remember an incident when I wished I had said no but didn't have the confidence to argue with the nurse at the time. It was the middle of the night, and finally, we were all sleeping soundly: my tiny daughter, my husband, and I. Then a busybody nurse came in and woke us all up, saying it was time to give my baby a bath. I protested, as the baby was sleeping and I didn't want to wake her up. The nurse insisted she had to stay on schedule. I reluctantly agreed and woke my sleeping angel. The nurse also didn't want my husband to go with her when she bathed the baby. This we did insist on, and he groggily followed her and watched my screaming baby have a bath in the middle of the night. I was deeply bothered by this interruption of our valuable and limited rest. The next day, I asked the day nurse about this disturbance. She said it would have been no problem to wait until the next morning for the baby to have a bath. Learn from this. You are the parent. If something doesn't feel right, say no.

While at the hospital, you will be provided with pain medication, stool softeners, and a squirt bottle for sanitizing after you use the bathroom. You will be bleeding a lot and just want to rest. You will be ready to take a shower the second day. Take it nice and slow, and it will feel great. Get rid of the crusty sweat, blood, and blah feeling. Have comfortable, loose clothing to change into. (Flannel pajamas are my favorite.) Because of your excessive bleeding, you will probably ruin any underwear you bring, so pack old, stretched-out maternity panties that you will be happy to throw away. Additionally, you will need the excessively big pads the hospital provides, which are so ridiculously large they will stick out of your underwear at all edges. Your bleeding will ease up after twenty-four hours or so, and you can kiss those silly pads good-bye and start using your regular maxi pads. You will be ready and happy to bring your new baby home. The car ride home is surreal. You have a new tiny passenger! The last time you rode in this car, that baby wasn't there—now she is! What?

CHAPTER 12

Home from the Hospital

> I just landed on my butt-head.
> —E., Age Three

For the first several days after you and Baby get home from the hospital, you're in a bit of a fog. You are very sore, extremely tired, and completely happy. You have a new pretty young thing to love![74] ♪ If your bedroom is upstairs, you will be confined up there for a few days, as you will need to rest and avoid stairs to let your perineum heal properly; that's especially important if you had stitches. You will be nursing, changing baby, and sleeping, and that's about it.

What you will need from visiting friends or family is help keeping the house in order. A mom/wife usually runs the house, and when a mom/wife is out of commission, the household may explode. If people want to help, let them do the laundry, housekeeping, and cooking. If people want to bring you something, ask for food! You will be hungry but will not be able to cook. Dad will appreciate gifts of food as well, because he'll also be exhausted. Cooked casseroles, chili, fresh ingredients for sandwiches, and gift cards for takeout/delivery will be greatly appreciated. You'll want to keep visits from guests short and sweet. You are too tired to host or entertain. You need to stay in your pajamas and rest with Baby. Dad's job will be to take care of you, feed you, bring you water, bring you ice pads, and to let you get rest.

---

74 "P.Y.T. (Pretty Young Thing)," Michael Jackson, *Thriller*, 1983, Epic Records.

You will be on painkillers for the first few days—acetaminophen and ibuprofen can be greatly effective, and it's usually OK to take both, if needed. By alternating medications, you'll have both types in your system, which will help you cope. Your midwife or nurse will help you get your medication schedule sorted out. Stool softeners are also recommended at first. The hospital will provide you with some for your stay, but you'll want to continue these when you get home for the first couple of days. You will need squirt bottles in all bathrooms so you can rinse your sore bottom after using the toilet. Pat gently to dry. You will need an ample supply of extra-long maxi pads and some frozen into ice pads. You will also need someone helpful to get them for you from the freezer (hello, Husband). Sitz baths may be soothing for those without stitches, but if you do have stitches, do not take baths of any kind for six weeks; you could get an infection in that area, which is extremely painful (yes, it happened to me with my first). Showers are completely OK, and they feel so nice. Hint: a nozzle with a long hose is very helpful to rinse hard-to-reach areas.

Ideally, I recommend that Baby sleep in your bedroom for the first four months. Set up a bassinet/playpen right next to your bed and a comfortable chair nearby. You will want to hear your baby breathing next to you at night. Even if you are asleep—trust me—if she needs you, you will hear her. If your baby coughs or starts to spit up, you can quickly pick her up to burp her and wipe away the spit up. When she wakes for yet another night feeding, you are right there to pick her up and feed her in the cozy rocking chair.

Have a convenient changing setup in your bedroom, too. Just a simple change pad that you can grab and put on your bed will work fine. Keep a basket of diapers, diaper cream, and wipes readily available. You don't want to be fumbling around for items in the dark when your little one is crying from hunger.

After the first few days, you can start venturing downstairs. It feels so liberating! My midwives always advised me to go up and down the stairs no more than the number of days old the baby was:[75] if she's three days old, then only three trips that day, for instance. See

---

75 Claudette Leduc, RM, and Lisa Weston, RM

chapter 10, "Care of Your Body after Birth," for my special postnatal stair-climbing strategy. Now you're ready to start enjoying your time with your baby. Hey—you're off work, you have a new tiny person in your life, this is new, and this is going to be good!

CHAPTER 13

Breastfeeding

Mommy, you'd better feed him
now, with your nipples.
—T., Age Six

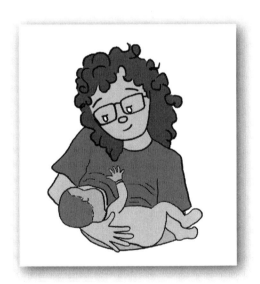

By now we've all heard that breastfeeding can have remarkable health benefits for Baby and Mom. Numerous studies suggest the baby winds up healthier and smarter; the research is undisputed.[76]

---

76 http://www.babycenter.com/0_how-breastfeeding-benefits-you-and-your-

It's also great for Mom—breastfeeding helps get your tummy back in shape as many calories are used to make milk (calories that could have been left sitting on your body as fat, instead wind up being consumed by your baby). Additionally, your body naturally contracts the uterus as your baby nurses, which helps your tummy shrink. Breastfeeding can reduce your chance of breast cancer later in life.[77] What you may not know about breastfeeding is the indescribable feeling that accompanies it. This is truly a special experience for you both. Nothing could bring you closer. Breastfeeding should be comfortable and relaxed for mother and baby, and it should happen as often and as much as the baby wants. When you wonder, "How can the baby possibly be hungry again? He just ate!" the answer is he just is; he loves and needs your milk!

I love breastfeeding. I love the connection you feel with the baby. The bond a mother and baby develop during this special time is long lasting and truly special. You feel so in tune and cuddly with your little one; you are both warm and snuggled together. Your baby looks at you with gratitude and comfort. Your baby's favorite spot will be in your arms, suckling your breast. It is another magical gift of nature that, one, your body can actually grow a real live human being inside of it and, two, it can produce a lovely, nutritious, and delicious food for this tiny little human being. The female body is so clever.

Breastfeeding is extremely convenient. You have no bottles to prepare or formula to pour in the middle of the night: all you have to do is lift up your shirt and dinner is ready. There is no need to pile bottles of milk in a cooler to take on the road when you already have to pack a million other things. Wherever you go, your milk is always fresh and ready and well packed…or well stacked.

I know some women find breastfeeding difficult. I was very lucky to have an easy time of it with my babies. Your midwives and the nurses at the hospital will help you get started. I encourage you to stick with it and work through the challenges if you have them. The rewards are significant. If you need further help, see a lactation consultant. In many communities, these experts lead free breastfeeding clinics; ask

baby_8910.bc

77 http://www.scientificamerican.com/article/breastfeeding-benefits-mothers/

your family doctor or local public health nurse for more information. I went to one of these sessions, and found it helpful and supportive. Many different moms were bonding and sharing breastfeeding strategies and stories.

The key to successful breastfeeding is a good latch. My midwives, Claudette Leduc and Lisa Weston, from Sages-Femmes Rouge Valley Midwives, taught me well. A good latch is when the baby's mouth is wide open, and the nipple is placed as far in as possible, pointing toward the roof of the baby's mouth. The baby's lips should be turned slightly upward on the breast, flanged (like a fish). Baby should be looking up at you, her chin up slightly, to open up her throat (helpful for swallowing). Her chin will be on the breast, which will massage the ducts, encouraging more milk to come. Holding your baby properly can also help you establish a good latch. It is important to face the baby's entire body toward your body. You should be belly to belly. You don't want her to have to turn her face to reach your nipple. You also need to pull Baby's body right up close to you. Tuck her bottom snugly to the side of your belly to be sure her little nose is lifted slightly up from the breast so she can breathe easily.

Start breastfeeding as soon as your baby wants to, right after giving birth. You will be holding your new, fresh baby skin to skin. Your baby will be ready to nurse within minutes. Don't believe the common misconception that your baby won't get enough milk for the first few days until your milk comes in. That is simply not true. (You will know when your milk comes in because your breasts will dramatically increase in size and weight.) There is no need to feed your baby formula during this time. That is actually detrimental to your breastfeeding success. When your baby is nursing for the first few days and your breasts haven't filled up with milk yet, your baby is still getting the nourishment she needs. Your breasts are producing liquid called colostrum that's full of antibodies that will help protect and build your baby's immune system. This is good stuff! Don't let your baby miss it.

Find a way to make yourself completely comfortable when breastfeeding. Lean back on your chair, prop Baby up with your nursing pillow, and completely relax. (If the nursing pillow was vomited on and is in the laundry, two regular pillows propped up like a *V* from your arms toward your lap will work as a satisfactory substitute.) Use this interlude to catch your breath and mellow out while your baby is blissfully suckling away, completely comfortable and relaxed.

Babies often fall asleep when breastfeeding before they are actually finished. The simple act of wiggling your nipple can get your baby sucking again so he gets the milk he needs before he drifts off to dreamland. I always let my babies fall asleep while nursing. It is the most natural thing to happen, so don't fight it. When Baby is asleep, his limbs are floppy, and the nipple falls out of his mouth. Gently burp him and lay him down for a peaceful nap.

The pattern for breastfeeding is very often—especially at first. I always breastfed on demand—whenever my baby wanted milk, I gave it to him for as much and as long as he wanted. I found myself breastfeeding every two hours twenty-four hours a day for a while. There is no schedule for the first bit; you just have to follow Baby's lead. During the early, newborn phase, the baby is the boss. What he wants goes! It eases up as the baby gets older and can drink more at one feeding. I always breastfed only one side (one breast) per feeding to ensure that the baby got the hind milk—the milk that contains the most fat. This milk is the most filling, so it will satiate the baby for longer, and it is good for brain development.[78] With each feeding, switch breasts. I could always tell which breast I was on because it would feel fuller. If you can't tell or have trouble keeping track, try a physical reminder such as a tissue in the bra of the breast just finished.[79] My babies were all very chubby babies and giving them the hind milk was probably one reason for that. Chubby babies are healthy babies. And not to mention, they are cute babies! (But then again, aren't all babies cute?)

Breastfeeding in public is a nonissue. It is now socially accepted, and moms do it, pretty much, everywhere. To maintain your privacy, invest in a good nursing shawl. It goes around your neck so the cover stays in place, even when babies are squirmy and flailing about. Good nursing shawls have a piece of moldable wire inside at the top, so there's a nice gap for ventilation and for Mom to look down and Baby

78 https://www.llli.org/faq/foremilk.html
79 Shalimar Santos-Comia, RN and mom

to look up. If you forgot your nursing shawl and are out and about, tuck a receiving blanket under your bra strap to help hold the blanket in place. Just throwing the fabric over your shoulder does not work so well: it falls off or Baby pulls it off, and you end up giving people a show! Another handy shawl substitute is a cardigan sweater or zip sweatshirt worn backward, with the opposite sleeve tucked in on the breastfeeding side. That will hold the sweater in place and amply conceal your breast and your baby from prying eyes. If you don't feel comfortable breastfeeding in public, look for a private nursing area wherever you are. Most public spaces have a small office, room, or corner where you can nurse your baby, alone. In my experience, when asked for this, people are very accommodating.

Leaky breasts prompt many women to start wearing a nursing bra to bed. I just couldn't do it! My girls needed to be free in the night! I hated the tight feeling of a bra around my chest when I was sleeping, and I felt that my nipples and breasts wanted to breathe so I slept braless. After a series of leaky-milk episodes (one breast will squirt like a hose when the baby begins sucking on the other and the milk is being "let down"—when the milk drops into the breast, and you feel a lot of pressure all of a sudden) and multiple nocturnal shirt changes, I figured out a solution. Keep a clean receiving blanket by the nursing pillow. When you are feeding the baby without a bra, just pull up your shirt and expose both breasts. Bunch up a section of the receiving blanket and cover your nonnursing nipple. The receiving blanket can absorb the excess milk, and your pajama shirt can stay dry. This makes for a nice, dry sleep and a little less laundry.

If your baby develops a little milk blister on her lip, don't be alarmed. It's from the friction of nursing and will dry up and fall off. It may come back again, but in my experience, the blisters don't bother the baby; and after several months she won't get them anymore.

Some women worry that breast milk isn't enough for the baby. What if the baby needs more nutrition—or more milk? From my experience, your breast milk is plenty and more. Your body is constantly producing milk. You don't run out. The more the baby suckles, the more milk you will make. In fact, if you decide to supplement with formula, you will disrupt Mother Nature's law of supply and demand.

The less time the baby is suckling, the less milk your breasts produce. Just keep eating and drinking, and you will keep producing. Yum for Mommy and Baby!

Mastitis, also known as a breast infection, is common for nursing mothers and is extremely painful. Some women are prone to them, some not at all. I was one of the unlucky ones—with my second and fourth newborns, I suffered bothersome mastitis. I also figured out how to prevent it from coming back. Mastitis starts with a clogged milk duct. You can feel a large, hard mass in your breast; sometimes it extends very high into your chest or underarms in bead-like strings or a round or solid tube-shape. It makes your breast feel very heavy and sore. Untreated, the condition can be extremely painful and you can develop a fever and feel utterly ill. In that case, your doctor will probably prescribe a round of antibiotics. (Sometimes they're necessary but are not great for you or the nursing baby.)

You can take natural steps to prevent mastitis. If you feel soreness in a breast or notice it is an odd shape and heavier than usual, you could have a clogged milk duct. Act *now* to prevent it from becoming infected. This is what to do:

1. Empty the breast.
   - Nurse and/or pump; get it all out.
   - A family doctor explained to me that the breast ideally should be completely empty after a feeding, as bacteria from the baby's mouth can work its way into the breast and can breed and hang out in there if there is extra milk sitting around. Sometimes nursing the baby doesn't empty you completely, so pumping or manually expressing could be helpful to clear out the milk.[80] I couldn't be bothered to pump after every feeding, but I manually expressed milk right afterward each time. After nursing, I would simply squeeze my areola (the dark area encircling the nipple)

---

80 http://www.mayoclinic.org/diseases-conditions/mastitis/basics/causes/con-20026633

and squirt out a little bit of milk. I found this action was enough to cleanse the breast. I call it the "nurse and squirt" approach. I used it regularly, especially after healing from a breast infection, and I think it helped.

2. Massage the breast.
   - By massage, I don't mean a gentle, lovely, relaxing rub. I mean a vigorous movement and shaking of the breast. It hurts. You will need to do some deep breathing to get through it, but it works to unclog the breast and help prevent infection (which is much worse).
   - To massage the breast effectively, cup the breast with one hand and move it in fast circles as big as you can go. Repeat this often throughout the day. It hurts, so bite your lip and take deep breaths. Additionally, poke and prod the lumpy and sore part of the breast. Use your fingers to try to break up the clog and press to "push" the clog out of the breast.
   - When you massage, use strong force. Really give the breast a workout; massage deeply and press hard to attempt to move any lumps of milk along. (See above.) You can press right into your armpits. Go from the back of the breast toward the nipple and express milk, just like milking a cow. Manually squeeze milk out and make sure your breasts are nice and soft.

3. Apply heat.
   - I'm not talking a nice warm compress here; I'm talking *hot*, as hot as you can handle. I use fabric heating/cooling compresses filled with flaxseeds. These mold nicely to your shape and can be reheated repeatedly. Keep the heat on almost constantly for the entire day. Hot compresses are great. They help with the pain, and they open up the milk ducts and keep things flowing. Put them on tight up against the sore area for a long time, repeatedly. Imagine you are trying to melt the clogged milk. Watch you don't burn your skin. Place the heat on top of a layer of clothing to prevent burns.

Those are my three steps for stopping a clogged milk duct from becoming full-blown mastitis. Repeat these steps constantly, all day. Your breast should feel noticeably better the next day.

If you can, see a naturopathic doctor and try acupuncture.[81] These methods may help prevent the need for antibiotics. But if you do get mastitis, see your doctor and take your antibiotics as directed; the drugs he prescribes will be breastfeeding-safe. You can take probiotic supplements (i.e., acidophilus) or eat lots of yogurt to replenish your good bacteria.

Mastitis is known for reoccurring. Prevention is key. Consider these additional preventive steps:

- Keep nursing your baby and pumping if needed. Keep that milk moving.
- See a naturopathic doctor about vitamins and herbs that can boost the immune system and help the body fight infection.[82]
- You may also want to get acupuncture to keep the lymphatic system flowing. It helped me.
- Hot showers where you massage your breasts daily also help.[83]
- Taking lecithin capsules may help make the milk less sticky, hence less apt to cause the clogging that can lead to infection.[84]
- Try feeding Baby in different positions to change up where the milk is draining from, to really empty out all parts of the breast.

You want to avoid mastitis—the pain can be debilitating. Don't let this annoying problem get in the way of your feeding your baby!

At approximately four months, your baby may start biting you during breastfeeding. It actually hurts! Her little jaws clamp down on your nipple. To stop her, I simply looked her in the eye and firmly said no or "No biting." I also developed a feeling for when the baby was about to bite down, and before she could, I would place my finger and thumb

---

81 Dr. Lisa Doran, naturopathic doctor
82 Dr. Lisa Doran, naturopathic doctor
83 Ibid.
84 http://www.breastfeedinginc.ca/content.php?pagename=doc-BD-M

on the baby's chin and pull her mouth open. I learned to do it quickly and in a way that wouldn't separate her from the breast but it would prevent the bite.

For some babies, this biting phase passes quickly. With my first three, it was always over well before they got teeth. (Thank goodness!) However, my last baby, little Maxwell, went through a trying phase during nursing: he was teething and his gums hurt, and he bit my nipples *hard*! Ouch! The trick I came up with: if he was in a biting mood (he was cranky, his teeth hurt, he was feeling playful, or he was not very hungry), then I would make sure his head was close to my breast. I figured out that if he was about to bite, his head would pull away slightly, but with his head pushed right up close and his mouth wide over the nipple, he was unable to bite. If I notice him squirming back from my close hold, I would quickly slip my nipple out of his mouth before he was able to chomp down. I figured out a rhythm. Get ready with your thumb in the bend of his chin in case you don't pull your nipple out of his mouth in time. Just watch out for the twist, pull, and bite trick! When something nabs your baby's wandering attention, and her little eyes follow, oops and ouch! These little nibbles are painful, but for me anyway, the pluses of breastfeeding outweigh the pain. Remember, babies grow out of it. Continue saying no in a firm voice when it happens. Maxwell's bad biting phase lasted about a month.

CHAPTER 14

Pumping Breast Milk

> How can one mommy love one
> baby so incredibly much?
> —Me

I wanted my babies to get the benefits from breast milk for as long as possible. Additionally, it seemed to me that since I was producing such a valuable commodity, I should capitalize on this special resource by pumping and freezing it for later. So, with each baby, I pumped and froze milk once a day. When I had to go back to work after a year of maternity leave and breastfeeding on demand, I gave my babies bottles and sippy cups of thawed breast milk to keep the health bonuses flowing. My babies drank only breast milk until they were approximately eighteen months old. That's when the frozen breast milk ran out and when I weaned them completely.

I developed a system for this process—it's not as simple as just pumping and freezing. You need to take a few steps to preserve the milk in the best possible condition. First of all, get a deep chest freezer that cools to approximately -20°C. A side-by-side or small fridge freezer won't keep the milk usable for as long.[85] In a deep chest freezer, breast milk stays good for up to one year. I labeled the bags by month and then stored them in numbered shoe boxes so we would use up the oldest milk first. Be sure to purchase the correct storage

---

85 www.medela.ca

bags for breast milk. These are BPA-free and seal airtight to prevent spillage.

You'll find many varieties of breast pumps on the market. I used a small electric one, as I only pumped once a day. Your choice may depend on how often you plan to pump. I purchased four-ounce glass bottles to use with the pump and disposed of the plastic bottle sold with it. Standard bottles have the correct size opening. Be sure to wash the parts of the pump separately. When I first started using the pump, I left the pieces intact and washed it in the dishwasher (top rack). Then I saw that black mold was growing inside it! Argh! So each part needs to be removed for correct cleaning and drying. You can also sterilize the parts by boiling them for five minutes. I did that from time to time. If you don't plan to give the pumped milk to your baby until after he is six months old, you don't need to sterilize it with each use. Washing it correctly is sufficient. By six months babies begin to eat solid food, and they are putting toys and random items in their mouths. In other words, their immune systems are getting stronger.

I started pumping right away, as soon as my milk came in, which typically happens two to three days after giving birth. You will feel extremely engorged and in pain with huge, swollen breasts. Pumping can help relieve this pressure. I gradually pumped less often as the engorgement went away and my breasts began to feel better.

I always pumped at the same time each day. A regular schedule trains your body to produce enough milk for the pumping session. For me, early in the morning, right after breakfast, worked well, because then it was done, and I didn't have to worry about it for the rest of the day. Pumping is most efficient directly after nursing. So I would nurse the baby with one breast, and when he was finished and settled, I would pump the other one: the milk would be in the breast and ready to go. I kept pumping until the milk stopped coming or my bottle was full. If the milk stops or significantly slows, and you feel your breast is not yet empty, you can encourage more milk to come by massaging the breast while pumping. I found it especially helpful to simply take a finger and press firmly down in one spot so more milk would be pushed out; then I'd move to another spot until the breast was empty. Often the lower half of the breast needed this assist, which makes sense: simple gravity pulls the milk down to the underside of the breast where it can be harder for the pump to pull it back up and out. I could have pumped even more than I did, because production increases the more you do, but I decided one small bottle of milk a day was enough. I continued for almost a year, so when I was finished I had almost 365 bags of milk (give or take!) because I pumped once a day.

Watch out for sour milk! An important note about storing breast milk is that some women produce an enzyme that makes milk taste sour when it is frozen and thawed. Mothers (me included) usually discover that when the baby doesn't appear to like the taste. The enzyme doesn't make the milk harmful, but the baby won't want to consume it.[86] My sister found this out the hard way, forfeiting an entire useless freezer-full of breast milk. So taste-test one bag of thawed milk first to see if it contains this problematic enzyme. The good news: you can do something about it! Scalding the milk before freezing it will kill the enzyme and eliminate the problem. This information is in the fine print that comes with the breast pump, but few people actually bother to read it (www.medela.ca).

Here's how to scald the milk (it's actually pretty easy). Get a small pot and put it on the burner, empty, at maximum temperature. Leave it there a few seconds, until you know it's warming up. Then pour your freshly squeezed breast milk in. Watch the milk constantly, as this next step only takes a few seconds—maybe twenty. As soon as the milk bubbles, remove it from the heat. Be ready; it bubbles quickly. (If you wait too long, and it's been bubbling for a while, then the milk will turn a sad gray color; and will need to be dumped out with a huge sigh. I couldn't feed my baby sad, gray milk.)

As soon as you remove it from the heat, pour the milk into a fresh glass bottle and put a glass lid on top. (I used a small glass bowl as a lid.) This keeps the steam in so all the water doesn't end up evaporating from the milk. Don't use plastic, as heated plastic can leach toxins into your pure, wonderful milk. Set the milk on the counter or in the fridge until it cools. When it is cool, stir it thoroughly with a small

---

86 www.medela.ca

spoon to mix the healthy fat back in (otherwise the fat rises to the top and sticks to the sides of the bottle). Next, pour the liquid into a proper breast milk storage bag, write the date on it, and place it in the deep chest freezer.

It's amazing how quickly your freezer will completely fill up with breast milk. You need an organized, compact storage system to maximize the limited space. Additionally, you'll want to use up the oldest milk first, so keep the date-labeled bags of milk in labeled shoe boxes. When you place a bag of milk inside a box, put it on top of the others; the bags will take one another's shape so you can fit more in. If you stand them up, they will freeze in a formation that takes up too much space. Frozen breast milk is such a nice prize to take out later and give your baby—the special gift of Mommy's milk.

MY BREAST MILK PUMPING SYSTEM STEP-BY-STEP

1. Pump at the same time each day, directly after nursing.
2. After pumping, scald the milk (if it contains the enzyme making it sour when thawed).
   a) Place an empty pot on a stove burner, over high heat.
   b) After a few seconds, pour the fresh breast milk in the pot.
   c) Watch the milk constantly.
   d) When it begins to bubble, remove it from the heat.
   e) Pour it into a glass bottle.
   f) Place glass lid on top.
   g) Allow it to cool.
   h) Stir with a small spoon to remix the healthy fat.
3. Pour into a breast milk storage bag.
4. Label by month.
5. Place in a deep chest freezer in numbered shoe boxes.
6. Clean breast pump correctly by separating all parts and washing individually.
7. To use milk, remove from freezer and thaw in fridge or in a cup of cold water.

Pumping breast milk is a bit of a chore, but you will get into a rhythm, and it becomes part of your routine. I did it daily for the majority of the first year with each baby. When is it time to stop pumping? When a) your freezer is stuffed full, b) you are sick of it, or c) one to two months before you return to work. Ceasing now gives your body a gradual letdown from producing so much milk before you're back at the office. When you do go back, it's an amazing feeling to know your baby will still be drinking your healthful, beautiful breast milk and is still getting all that goodness, even when you're not there.

Note: if you go on an overnight getaway (woo-hoo! good for you), pumping gets problematic. You can bring your pump and use it, but you can't scald and freeze the milk. Your options:

a. Don't pump while on vacation
   - Your breasts will be engorged at first, as they are used to making an extra bottle of milk each day, causing discomfort. Then with time, your body adjusts, but when you resume pumping, it takes a while to get the extra milk back up and running. It is doable; it will just take a gradual readjustment once you're home.
b. Pump and dump
   - What a waste! I cringe to see the milk my body has worked to make and I've worked to expel just go down the drain. ☹
c. Pump and feed breast milk to toddler
   - This is a great option (my favorite). Your body continues its regimen of producing extra milk, and it doesn't go to waste. It's healthy for your toddler; just put it in a sippy cup and call it special Trip Milk.
d. Pump, refrigerate, and take home
   - This option is risky, as milk could spoil
   - May be cumbersome, extra bag (cooler) to carry and pack
   - Must be diligent about keeping ice packs cold, need access to a freezer

CHAPTER 15

Offering a Bottle to a Breastfed Baby

I need milk now, or else I'm going to get old.
—P., AGE FOUR

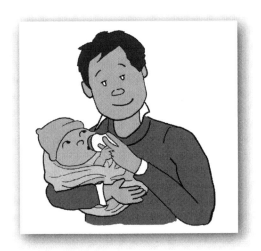

There is no real need to give an exclusively breastfed baby a bottle. Some moms feel obligated to have their babies drinking out of a bottle (society expectations? Grandma's way?), but it's simply not necessary. You can just skip the bottle and go right to a sippy cup. My babies all loved the breast and at first hated the bottle, especially while they were still small infants. I waited until they were six months old, and then presented the bottle to them in a different way. I decided to offer them the bottle at six months, to begin to give them another method of getting milk. My intention was to prepare them to be a bit more independent for when we were out and about, or if I wanted to take the dog for a walk, and could then leave them with daddy and a bottle. Rather than cuddle them in my arms and push the bottle into their mouth (with them, that would never work!), I gave it to them while they sat in the high chair and let them explore it on their own, just like I would give them a new food to try. I served the bottled breast milk cold so my baby would get used to it at that temperature.[87] That made travel much easier, free of the need for bottle-warming or the chance of wasting breast milk through reheating and spoiling. (You can't reheat milk twice).

My babies would sip at the bottle but not guzzle. It was their choice, not a struggle. If they wanted to drink a lot, they wanted me. To me, this was just fine! I often put water in the bottle instead of milk, since babies trying out this new type of nipple will waste a lot by spilling, spitting, dribbling, or just not drinking it all. Playing and experimenting with the bottle is how my babies learned to drink from it—on their own terms, without pressure or tension. In the eleventh month of maternity leave when you're preparing to return to work, keep offering your baby the bottle or sippy cup. He will learn to drink from it, and by the time you're at the office, he'll know how to drink what he needs while you are away. When you're with him, he doesn't need to drink from other sources and most likely won't. Your baby will get what he needs, so don't worry about it!

If you need to have your baby on a bottle earlier but still want to breastfeed as well, you'll have to introduce the Other Nipple very early in her life; otherwise, you'll be met with resistance! One tip: babies may more readily accept a bottle from someone other than Mom (Dad, Grandma, an aunt, or a nanny). If Mom is holding him and offering the bottle, he won't see the point. Babies know the milk is right there in those breasts! Additionally, for some bottle-fed babies, the issue of "nipple confusion" is real: they have trouble going back to the breast if you introduce the bottle too early. Bringing on the bottle

87 Shalimar Santos-Comia, RN and mom

(or not) is a decision you'll have to make and then "go with"; and your baby will figure out a system that works best. See the next chapter for information and tips for using both feeding methods in the same time frame.

Note: Once your baby starts walking, don't let him walk around with a glass bottle. These can smash (it happened with Terrek, twice). Now is an excellent time to switch to a sippy cup.

CHAPTER 16

Bottle- and Breastfeeding Together

> I'm going to be a bad raccoon that likes everybody.
> —E., AGE THREE

Some moms like the flexibility of being able to both breastfeed and bottle-feed right from the get-go. Perhaps they anticipate needing to return to work early, perhaps Daddy wants to take a turn feeding, or maybe Mom would like to be able to leave Baby with Grandma and run errands for a while. While I didn't use dual feeding with my kids, I spoke with a mom of three, Yvette Tsang, who developed a stellar plan for doing just that.

Yvette had to go back to work a few months after the birth, so she needed to prepare her baby girl but also wanted to give her (and enjoy) the benefits of breastfeeding. She found a way that her baby could have her milk and drink it, too—by breastfeeding and bottle-feeding (with pumped breast milk) interchangeably. While it's a challenge when the baby prefers the breast and resists the bottle, Yvette appreciated being able to use both methods. She loved the cozy closeness of breastfeeding, but also the ability to sleep five hours while her husband took over one of the nightly feedings. (I have to admit, this does sound heavenly!) Time was another issue. When you have only one baby, you have every waking minute to spend breastfeeding your baby if need be. But when her third baby was born, Yvette had a busy household with a three-year-old and a six-year-old who needed her, too.

So how did she do it? The key, she found, is to start with the bottle early. Breastfeed as soon as possible after the birth; then, within the first week, start pumping and introduce the bottle. Introduce it very gently the first time, Yvette suggests. The baby may not take to it right away, but don't force it, she says; just give the breast and try again tomorrow.

An effective strategy to introduce the bottle for the first time: Gently place the nipple in the baby's mouth. Never force it in. Let the baby play with the nipple. Squeeze the bottle's nipple so that some milk is dripping out of the nipple and the baby can taste and smell that her favorite food is there, only presented in a different way. Tease the baby a little by pulling the nipple away. This will encourage the baby to reach for the nipple and suck harder to get the nipple to come back. Let the baby bite and chew on the nipple. Rub the nipple on her lips until she latches on. Let her feel the nipple. Pull it gently out and push it gently back in. Move the nipple in and out of her mouth very slowly to get the baby to latch and hold on to the nipple. It might take her a while to get the hang of it, but continue this.

Yvette's baby caught on after about a week of this process, although a baby may never latch on as smoothly or enthusiastically as she latches onto the breast. Yvette found that with the bottle, her baby had difficulty controlling the flow, and a lot of milk dribbled and spilled. She recommends continuing to feed regularly with the breast; then, one or two times a day, use the bottle full of freshly pumped breast milk so the baby becomes familiar with both.

Breast and bottle-feeding together requires planning and fore-sight about timing. When your baby is feeding every two to three hours, Yvette points out, you need to think ahead to the next feeding. Will you be using the breast or the bottle? You don't want to pump if you'll need your breasts to be full for the next session. You'll need to estimate, and if you plan on breastfeeding soon, don't pump all the milk out. Sometimes the baby will feed more often, and in that case, even when you plan very carefully, it might not always work out. That's why Yvette recommends always having two extra bottles of breast milk in the fridge. You will get into a rhythm where you are breastfeeding or pumping every two or three hours. And again, the more you pump, the more milk your body will make.

Yvette warmed her bottles of breast milk by using boiling water. If boiling the water takes too long for your impatient baby, consider getting an electric water heater and warmer (Yvette has one of these!), which provide boiling water at the touch of a button. They're available in small-appliance sections of department stores and are handy for quick tea and coffee, too. To warm the milk, place boiling water in a container slightly larger than the bottle and place the bottle full of cold breast milk inside. Let it sit a few minutes. Test the milk on your wrist to ensure that it's not too hot or cold; the same temperature as your body is just right, meaning you really shouldn't feel anything on your wrist. When out and about, Yvette carried cold breast milk in an insulated lunch bag with an ice pack, plus an insulated thermos full of boiling water and her container. That way, her baby could have nice warm breast milk wherever they went.

Yvette recommends a dual breast pump (two pumps included, one for each breast simultaneously) with a backpack, for pumping when you're back at work or on the go. She pumped on her lunch break, so her baby got breast milk for the first twelve months, which doctors recommend. At home in the evenings, you can feed with either breast or bottle. For the most part, with her feeding system, Yvette indeed found a way to get the convenience of the bottle and the benefits of the breast. With this system, it's the best of both worlds!

CHAPTER 17

Formula-Feeding

I'm so hungry All that's in my tummy is
only a speck, smaller than a germ.

—P., AGE FOUR

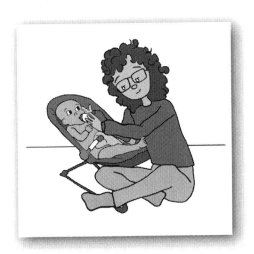

Sometimes, despite a mother's best efforts and intentions, breastfeeding just doesn't work. Her milk doesn't come in, or the baby just can't latch on correctly. Or perhaps Mom needs to go back to work too soon to rely on breastfeeding long term. If this is your situation, don't beat yourself up. You are still a good and wonderful mom! Baby formulas are always improving and now contain Omega fats and good bacteria (probiotics). Your baby will be just fine.

There is a big positive to bottle- and formula-feeding: you will have a lot more freedom. You won't be as tied to the baby as a breastfeeding mom is. If you need to get out and have a break, you will be able to leave Baby with Grandma, Dad, or a babysitter. Dad can even take over the night feedings one or two nights a week so Mom can actually get a good night's sleep![88]

Breastfeeding is heavily encouraged these days by doctors, midwives, and nurses, which can put a lot of pressure on you as a mom. Bottle-feeding is mentioned with a negative connotation.[89] But if you need to bottle-feed, please don't feel guilty or ashamed of your decision. You can't worry about what other people think. You have to do what is right and best for you and your baby. You may be told you will miss out on forming a crucial bond with your child, but that just isn't true. Be the best mom you can be, and you will still develop closeness and a long-lasting connection.[90]

Although I did not feed my babies formula, I have gathered a few tips on formula-feeding from excellent moms. Some use a combination of breast milk and formula, and some switch to formula after a certain amount of time. Some moms feed only with formula from day one. Whatever the reason, if formula is what works for you, embrace it! My sister-in-law Mary formula-fed three beautiful baby boys, and it was the perfect system for her family.

Formula comes in two versions: powder or liquid. While the powder is often more affordable, some moms find it has a chalky consistency and prefer the liquid.[91] Yet powder formula is easy to pack and store—you just add water. When my friend Maya was researching formula brands, nurses and doctors told her that all were comparable. However, with different formulas she noted subtle differences in her baby's poo and tummy aches or gas. She began charting the product ingredients, noting the varying effects on her baby, and hit on one the

---

88 Maya Castle, mom

89 Yvette Tsang, teacher and mom

90 Ibid.

91 Ellen Ryan-Chan, teacher and mom

baby handled best.[92] So you may also want to experiment with brands by at first buying only a small amount of each.

Many varieties of baby bottles are available. Some mothers find those with a valve system work well to prevent gas.[93] My friend Maya favors these; they require a few more steps for cleaning, she says, as the valve and parts must be disassembled and cleaned with a bottle brush, but "soon enough these steps become old habit and very simple to do."[94]

To disinfect the bottles and their various parts, boil them in a big pot of water for five minutes before each use. You can also purchase microwavable bottle sterilizers, but I am not a fan of heating plastic, so that would not be my first choice. Washing and sterilizing bottles two to three times a day is a chore,[95] but after your baby is three months old, using the top rack of the dishwasher is safe.[96] Prior to three months, your baby's immune system is very sensitive, and you don't want any germs entering her little system. Boiling the parts ensures that any bacteria or other contaminants are eliminated.

As for glass versus plastic, if you've read this far, you know I avoid chemicals at all costs and vote 100 percent for glass. Still, glass bottles are more difficult for babies to manipulate and learn to hold,[97] so you may want to use BPA-free plastic. Remember, don't let your toddler walk around with glass; as I related earlier, Terrek's dropped bottle ended up in a million shards of pointy glass around his feet. (Amazingly, he did not get a scratch.)

When you bottle-feed, you need to choose nipple flow speeds based on the baby's age. Nipples are sold with age recommendations on the packaging. My friend Maya found these didn't necessarily correspond to her baby's current feeding needs. She describes her son as a "voracious" eater who needed a higher flow rate than his age would

---

92 Maya Castle, mom
93 Mary Anne Pangilinan, mom
94 Maya Castle, mom
95 Yvette Tsang, teacher and mom
96 Maya Castle, mom
97 Ibid.

suggest. A very in-tune mother, she also noticed her baby was becoming frustrated while drinking and not getting enough milk at once. Or he would give up and fall asleep. She experimented with the next size up, and after some transition and training, her baby adjusted to the faster speed. It was a bit of a process: at first, he coughed and milk leaked from the corners of his mouth. She started out using the new nipple for only one feeding a day, and then gradually used it more as her baby got the hang of it.[98]

To ease nighttime feeding, my sister-in-law, Mary, set up a milk station in her bedroom, with a mini fridge and bottle warmer, so she wouldn't have to go down to the kitchen to prepare bottles in the middle of the night. You can also prepare the bottles before bed and put them in the fridge to grab and warm up quickly[99] while you change the baby's diaper. If you don't have a fridge near the bedrooms, you can premeasure powder formula and put it in the bottles, so all you have to do is add the water.[100] Or you can prepour the water and add the formula in the night.[101] Choose the system easiest for you. As for managing the dirty bottles at night, set up a bin or a bucket full of soapy water and let them soak for easy cleaning the next day.

While you can't premix formula for travel because it spoils quickly, there are some tips for transporting ingredients to make formula-on-the-go easier. Pack your cooler bag with premeasured water and premeasured formula in a divided container. (Each section holds a separate serving of formula). The container holds enough formula for three feedings and can fit into the mouth of the bottle, which minimizes spillage.[102] Pack hot or warm water in a thermos, or skip the warming step and teach your baby to enjoy formula made with room-temperature water.[103] He should get used to it quickly.

98 Maya Castle, mom
99 Mary Miller, teacher and mom
100 Ibid.
101 Maya Castle, mom
102 Ibid.
103 Shalimar Santos-Comia RN

Positioning your baby while bottle-feeding may also take some troubleshooting. While some moms and babies may gravitate to the traditional baby hold that resembles the close snuggle of breastfeeding, don't be afraid to experiment. For Maya, seating her baby in a bouncer chair or his car seat, facing her, worked best; she found he got less gassy and was able to drink more milk. She caressed her baby's cheek and looked into his eyes as he drank to promote that closeness that comes when a mommy is nourishing her child.[104]

---

104 Maya Castle, mom

CHAPTER 18

The Pacifier Debate

Mommy, these peejamies are not working
for me. They are making me not sleep.
—E., Age Three

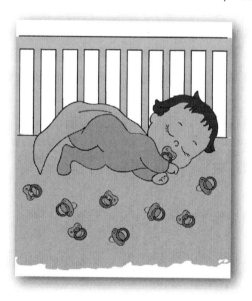

I have seen many babies over the years sucking madly away at their pacifiers and absolutely loving it! There must be some kind of magic with this clever little sucking device; however, my babies never used one. They didn't need to. It is my belief that if you are exclusively breastfeeding your baby and you breastfeed on demand, under regular circumstances there is no need for a pacifier. Babies have a strong natural instinct to suck. It settles them, fills their bellies, and keeps them close to Mama—all good things for them. If you are breastfeeding when your baby wants to breastfeed (frequently) and for as long as your baby wants (long), then this natural need is satisfied in the most natural way, by you. If your baby is a content baby who is usually happy and you are breastfeeding on demand, there is no need to introduce a pacifier. If a baby wants to suck, then the most natural thing for him to suck is the breast. As babies suck the breast, they are also constantly getting milk, making them nice and full and chubby so when they do nod off to sleep, they are satisfied.

Pacifiers, while offering lovely comfort and attachment while Baby is small, can be an extremely difficult habit to break. As babies turn into toddlers, they don't want to part with this comforting tool. And while a pacifier can help a baby nod off, babies often wake in the night screaming when their pacifiers fall out of their mouths because they are too little to pick it up and put it back in. When they are old enough to manipulate it with their hands, they still cry because they can't find it in the dark in their enormous crib. (And let's face it, we all know babies are thinking it's just nicer when Mom finds it for them anyway.) The result is a tired and disoriented mom stumbling into Baby's room and groping in the dark for a pacifier to pop back into Baby's mouth. Distraught Baby will be thankful and relieved to have his pacifier back and will quickly fall back to sleep, but then, lo and behold, the episode will repeat.

If your baby is having this problem, I have a brilliant tip for you from my friend Lisa, though it only works when Baby is old enough to pick up the pacifier and put it back into her mouth. When Lisa couldn't take the constant pacifier-searching in the middle of the night, she placed fifteen pacifiers around her baby in the crib so her baby could find at least one to reinsert during the night. This method actually resulted in Baby sleeping longer.[105]

I can see how, unlike babies who are breastfed on demand, bottle-feeders may indeed develop a need to suck. I have observed that

---

[105] Lisa Simms, mom

bottle-feeding is a much faster method of getting milk into Baby. The baby gets more with each mouthful and when the bottle is empty, the feeding is over. With the breast, the feeding can go on for longer periods, as the breast is rarely completely empty. (The milk machines are constantly producing more milk.) While I have not conducted scientific studies on the subject, my hunch is that babies who are bottle-fed may not get enough of the sucking sensation that meets an instinctive need at this time in their lives. From a physical standpoint, a pacifier makes sense.

If you are using a pacifier, please be careful not to give your baby one when she is actually hungry. If Baby is crying because she needs milk, give her milk! Don't shove a pacifier in her mouth and think, "She's fine; she can wait." There are few things sadder than a hungry baby who is not being listened to!

I've heard of other cases where pacifiers may be helpful. If your baby cries in the car, using a pacifier in the car can help quiet her[106] so you can drive safely and in peace. (Most very young babies fall asleep easily in the car, however.). Pacifiers reportedly help settle symptoms for some gassy babies.[107]

As with all aspects of being a mom, only you can decide. Whether or not your baby uses a pacifier, you will find your way, and you will make it work!

106 Ellen Ryan-Chan, teacher and mom
107 Lisa Simms, mom

CHAPTER 19

Diapering Baby

> Alert, alert! We've got a problem over here.
> —T., AGE FIVE

I n case you weren't aware, here's a heads-up: changing your baby's diaper will be a frequent pastime of yours for the next two to two-and-a-half years. What fun there is to come! Here is a bit of information to help you get the most out of your new hobby.

From the outset, of course, you will need to decide whether to use cloth or disposable diapers. I have used both: cloth for my first two children, disposables for my third and fourth. While disposables are certainly easier, cloth diapers are not actually that much work, or not as much as one might expect, anyway.

Cloth diapers are better for our planet. You reduce a huge amount of household waste by eliminating the dirty, plastic diapers from your garbage. Although cloth diapers do use up quite a bit of energy, with all the hot-water laundering, they are still the more environmentally friendly choice. Especially if you have a high-efficiency washing machine, and choose to hang dry the diapers. [108] Some jurisdictions allow you to put disposable diapers in the green bin to decompose with the food waste. I question this practice, as the plastics, bleaches, and harsh chemicals in diapers don't compost. They will just end up being crushed up and sitting in our soil. By choosing cloth, you also reduce the voluminous quantity

---

108 http://www.slate.com/articles/health_and_science/the_green_lantern/2008/03/should_my_baby_wear_huggies.html

of fossil fuels, paper products, bleach, and other chemicals needed to produce disposables—not to mention the cardboard boxes and plastic bags for packaging. Then there are the fossil fuels required to truck disposables from the factory to the store. Hands down, cloth diapers are the greener choice. Note: if you do choose disposable diapers, you may select all natural, unbleached diapers for a greener option.

Babies' bottoms are particular. Some babies get fewer diaper rashes with cloth diapers (my sons). They're soft on the skin, breathable, and free of the chemicals that disposables are made with. Some babies get fewer diaper rashes when using disposables (my daughter). Disposable diapers are drier and pull liquid away from your baby's skin. Cloth diapers are much more affordable. You spend a significant amount up front on the purchase of cloth diapers, but that's your only expense (besides the utility bills for the extra loads of laundry). When it comes time for potty training, cloth diapers can be helpful: your baby, uncomfortably wet and soggy when needing to be changed, may be more motivated to learn.

DECISION-MAKING TABLE: DIAPERS

ADVANTAGES

CLOTH DIAPERS	DISPOSABLE DIAPERS
☑ Greener; more environmentally friendly ☑ Less expensive ☑ Softer on Baby's bottom ☑ Easier to potty train with	☑ Easier ☑ Drier

DISADVANTAGES

CLOTH DIAPERS	DISPOSABLE DIAPERS
☒ Not good for night time ☒ Wetter ☒ More work (unless you get a diaper-laundering service)	☒ More expensive ☒ Not environmentally friendly

If you decide on cloth diapers, you can pick from many varieties. You can also choose traditional flat diapers that need to be folded (tricky for some, but I got the hang of it quickly). These go inside a cover. You do not use the old-fashioned pins at all, but a Velcro-fastened plastic cover. You can also choose the prefolded diapers that go inside a cover, or you can choose the all-in-ones with the liner attached. These are the easiest to use but also are the most expensive. Another option is diaper liners: soft, flushable layers you put inside the diaper, remove when dirty, and flush along with the waste. They help keep the diaper cleaner, especially when your child's poo changes after he starts eating solid foods. For further liquid-absorbency, try cloth diaper liner inserts. One hint regarding cloth: do not let an edge of clothing tuck into the diaper. If the diaper is wet, it will absorb the liquid and draw it out, soaking the outfit in pee.

With cloth diapers, you have yet another choice to make: wash them yourself or send out to a cleaning service. I never used the latter, but I'm sure it's a convenient choice!

Here's my system for washing cloth diapers. After changing Baby, throw the diapers in a bucket with a lid (available at the same place as cloth diapers are sold). You can throw them in dry or wet. Upstairs in the baby's room, by the changing station, I kept a dry bucket. I threw the diapers there and at the end of the day brought them downstairs to soak. Downstairs, I had a wet bucket where I'd soak used diapers in a solution of water and either white vinegar and Amaze (by Sunlight)[109] or Borax until laundry time. When your baby starts solid foods and his poo changes, you should shake it into the toilet and flush, or if you are using a liner, peel it out and flush. You may run into spillage or leakage at times and need to scrape or rinse the poo from the diaper before soaking. I kept an old toothbrush in the laundry tub for that. We also installed a hose with a powerful nozzle to squirt the diapers before soaking.

I washed the diapers every three days. First, I dumped most of the excess soaking solution (stinky by now) down the drain and threw the wet diapers and their dripping liquid into the washing machine. Start with a spin cycle to get rid of the excess liquid. Then switch to a

---

109 Oresta Korbutiak, mom

sanitize cycle (hot water). Be sure to use gentle laundry detergent free of scents and strong chemicals.

Actually, my old top-loader washing machine with an agitator did not have a sanitize cycle, so I just used a hot cycle. I think it actually worked better than my newer front-load machine, since after using the latter, I sometimes could still smell ammonia on the diapers and had to run them through another cycle. That's something to consider if you are purchasing a new washing machine.

As for drying, if the diapers feel wet and soggy when the wash is finished, run an additional spin cycle and then throw them in the dryer. Or hang them to dry outside, where (a bonus) the sun generally bleaches out the stains. You'll save on energy bills that way, though the diapers do take longer to dry; hanging them overnight and using the dryer a few minutes in the morning works, too.[110] When your cloth diapers are dry, fold them or just throw them in a basket in the closet. I always felt proud when my nice, clean diapers were ready to go for another round!

Important: cloth diapers are not a great solution for nighttime. Your baby can feel the wetness, which makes sleeping in them uncomfortable, and he will wake more frequently in the night. I found it best to use cloth diapers during the day and disposable diapers at night. Your baby sleeps better, meaning you also sleep better. Note: Huggies and Pampers both make a special overnight diaper that lasts twelve hours. I recommend these at about six to eight months. You'll know when your baby needs these if her diaper leaks in the night. They work for heavy wetters. I also found it much easier to use disposables when I was on the go. I didn't want to carry dirty cloth diapers around the mall or zoo in my already stuffed-to-the-max diaper bag. At the end of the day, it's nice to wrap your baby's bottom in soft, clean, gentle cloth at home.

A note about exploding poos: don't be alarmed, but breastfed babies have liquid-like poos that shoot out of their rear end with tremendous force. These poos have a way of shooting right out of the diaper and up the baby's back. This slimy mess ruins many outfits by staining them a puke-y mustardy color. It's inconvenient when you are

110 Amy Olar, teacher and mom

out and about, so always pack extra outfits and lots of baby wipes. The exploding poo stage will end after your baby starts on solid foods. In the meantime, upping the diaper size can sometimes contain the issue.

You may also try folding the back of the diaper to attempt to block the poo from shooting up your baby's back.[111] It may work occasionally, and cloth diapers may do a better job of this than do disposables. But in my experience, with four breastfed babies who all had healthy, expressive bowel movements, there is not much you can do to combat successfully the exploding poo phenomenon. Best to embrace it and come prepared! Extra diapers, extra clothes, many wipes, and a sense of humor are your best bets. Sometimes there is just no two ways about it: Baby needs a bath (no matter how much you wipe!).

Most baby registries suggest you purchase a fancy, tech-savvy diaper pail. These pails keep the dirty diapers in an airtight container to eliminate foul smells from your house. I had one of these, and I ended up throwing it in the garbage along with the stinky diapers. I found, and noticed every time I used mine or someone else's, that these diaper pails are not effective. Their purpose is to eliminate bad odors, yet they end up magnifying the foul smell by enclosing the stinky diapers in an airtight environment. The anaerobic bacteria are breeding! Therefore, whenever you brave the pail with the fancy opener to put in the next soiled diaper, a toxic, rancid, putrid, terrible, powerful stench escapes. It's just nasty! I still notice this whenever I'm in a public bathroom that offers one of these types of diaper pails. The smell is far worse than in a public bathroom where you toss the dirty diaper in the regular trash with the paper towels. The best solution for dirty diapers is a simple plastic grocery bag hung on the doorknob of your bathroom. Alternatively, use a simple bathroom garbage can without an airtight lid. Throw the entire bag in the garage or outdoor can when a) it's full or b) there is a stinky poo diaper going in. It's the best way to eliminate odors quickly. There's no need for the expensive diaper pail, with its inadvertent compounding of the problem.

With diaper changes comes the cream and powder decision. What kind of diaper cream works best? Well, the truth is, all babies' rear ends and skin are different. You will have to find what works best

---

111 Shalimar Santos-Comia, RN and mom

in your case. I like a zinc oxide cream that is light in consistency. With my two oldest boys, I used a lighter diaper cream and cornstarch baby powder (to help keep bottoms dry) with every change. My daughter had particularly sensitive skin, so I found her rear end did better with nothing at all.[112] Her skin needed air. My fourth baby also did best with nothing applied down there, until around eight months when he started getting diaper rashes, so I started using cream, and it helped. Watch your baby's posterior to figure out the best option for his skin. Some moms apply petroleum jelly; if you prefer not to use petroleum products, a layer of olive oil works just as well, creating a barrier against the moisture. Some moms prefer thicker diaper creams, and I know this type of cream is an old standby. It's very thick, but it has such a nice, familiar baby smell. See what works for your baby!

If your baby gets a rash-covered red bottom, that's diaper rash. It may start out with just a few pimply red speckles. The best way to heal diaper rash is to let your baby's rear end air out. Put her on a blanket, naked, and let the breeze do its magic. You can get a diaper cream with a stronger percentage of zinc oxide (40 percent). Wipes may sting a rash-covered rear, so you may want to use a warm, wet cloth (just water) to clean her when she has a rash. Be sure to dry her well before covering her back up again. If the diaper rash is not going away, you may need to consult your doctor and get a prescription cream. She could have a yeast infection, requiring an antifungal cream. Your doctor can also prescribe hydrocortisone cream, effective to banish diaper rash quickly; just apply a very thin layer at each application.

The actual diaper-changing process is pretty simple. Place a clean diaper under your baby's diapered bottom. Open the dirty diaper, wipe front to back with as many clean wipes as needed. Always go front to back so bacteria from the anus doesn't make its way to the penis or vagina. Always delve deeply into all chubby crevices. Dirty stuff is good at hiding in chubby folds of baby skin. Wipe them all out with wet wipes, and then pat gently dry with tissue. Don't skip this crucial step! As mentioned in chapter 23, "Fussy Baby," I find that patting with a tissue after wiping is the best-kept secret for preventing diaper rash[113].

112 Ellen Ryan-Chan, teacher and mom
113 Charmayne Richards, teacher and mom

Crevices are ample with baby girls. Be sure to gently separate the labia and wipe on the inside. Watch out for surprise peeing from baby boys! When the cold air hits the penis, urination can be a natural reflex. Treat the penis like a finger and wipe around it. There is no need to do anything different with an uncircumcised penis. Just wipe it clean.

After wiping is complete, fold the dirty diaper in half, and rest Baby's bottom on the clean side while drying him with the tissue. Apply cream or powder now (if using). Tip: keep your index fingernail short, so diaper cream does not accumulate under your nail. Better yet, use the back of your nail to scoop out some cream from the container so it can't make its way under the fingernail. Next, roll the dirty diaper up and pull it out from under the baby. The new diaper is already under the bottom in the ready position. Just fasten it up, and you're good to go!

When your baby reaches eight or nine months, she will begin the squirmy diaper-changing phase. Diaper changes get trickier! Baby will try to roll over, reach over there, grab that, and flip back again. It's a good idea to have some new toys or objects to keep the baby occupied while you change her. You'll have to embrace speed. Your baby doesn't have time to lie around all day on her back while you tend to her. Come on now, Mom! She has things to grab and objects to bite. You may want to consider placing a folded towel on the floor and forgo the change table. Your little monkey is coming into her own.

Another diaper-changing challenge pops up around this age (or younger). Your baby will discover that there are some new and interesting body parts under the diaper. He will love to grab these! This creates an extra job of washing your little one's hands (as well as yours) when you're done because you know where his little hands are headed next...directly into his mouth!

Whether you use cloth or disposable, be sure to change your baby's diaper often. It cuts down on diaper rash and keeps your baby more comfortable. It's not fair to be left to sit in one's own filth. Even if your brand's claims say the diaper is "absorbent enough to last twelve hours," that is meant for nighttime. During the day, it would be cruel to wait that long. Change diapers often. Embrace your new pastime by keeping your baby clean, dry, and happy!

CHAPTER 20

Cosleeping versus Crib Sleeping

> I want to stay with Mommy forever.
> —P., AGE THREE

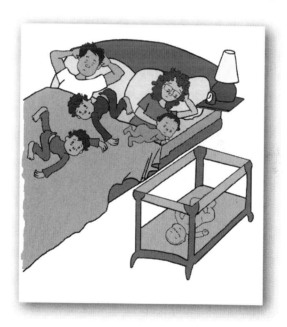

Few experiences are more gratifying than snuggling up with your newborn in your bed and drifting off to sleep together. You both sleep and enjoy being close and warm and cuddly. I was all for cosleeping after Terrek was born. He was my only child at the time, so all my time was for him. If he was sleepy, I lay down with him. I took him to bed with me at night, and we slept happily in each other's arms. I was in full support of this arrangement until one day on the phone my mom read me a newspaper article based on a coroner's report.[114] The report cited infant death rates due to suffocation from sleeping with adults. It really freaked me out. I decided nothing was worth that risk. Call me crazy, but if there is even a slight chance of my baby dying during a certain activity, then we are not going to engage in that activity!

My baby was five months old when I decided to stop cosleeping and to teach him to sleep on his own. He had become completely dependent on me to fall asleep. He would not go to sleep by himself. He screamed and screamed. I rubbed his tummy and sang to him for what seemed like hours. Breaking him from our nocturnal habit was extremely difficult. I learned from this experience that although sleeping together is lovely, it is easier and probably safer for the baby if the baby learns to sleep in the crib from day one. You still can have plenty of hours snuggling together and nursing in the rocking chair and days of holding each other as you go about life. But in my view, actual sleeping is best done separately.

In addition to creating a child who is parent-dependent in order to fall asleep, cosleeping presents several other problems. What do you do if you need to use the bathroom? You don't want your baby to roll off the bed while you're gone.

And that's just for starters. After a baby comes into a marriage, it can be hard to find time to spend on the marriage. That goes double if you decide to cosleep with your baby. Cosleeping certainly interferes with quality husband-and-wife time, by never allowing a chance for Mom and Dad to be alone together. Such time is important for a healthy marriage, so if you train your baby from the get-go to sleep alone, your marriage may thank you later.

Cosleeping can also keep you from getting things accomplished, as it means you are spending, pretty much, every moment with your baby, awake or asleep. You don't have a break per se. Nap times are

114 http://www.thestar.com/news/canada/2013/06/03/rate_of_infant_deaths_in_ unsafe_sleep_environments_unchanged_despite_increased_awareness_ontario_coro- ners_study.html, 03/20/2014

a great time to check things off your to-do list. In fact, quite often they're the *only times* to do that, let alone the things on the list! (Like take a shower, fold the laundry, check e-mail, do yoga, make soup…)

Another factor is the added sleep deprivation for Mom. When I was cosleeping with my baby, I found that I didn't fall into a deep sleep because I was always slightly aware of my baby. I kept one arm on my baby so I would know if he moved; I didn't want him rolling on the floor or for my husband's arm to fling on top of him. Never reaching deep sleep isn't helpful for moms who are already sleep deprived. Sleep is so valuable, especially during this early infant stage. Mom needs deep sleep to be able to function properly when she is (technically) awake.

If you decide to have more children, cosleeping presents even more of a problem. You just won't be able to nap with your baby when you have a toddler to attend to as well; you will be on toddler duty. Unless you have another adult with you daily and nightly, it just doesn't work. Your toddler will appreciate some one-on-one time with Mom while the baby is sleeping, time when you can bake cookies or paint a picture together.

For the first four months of my babies' lives, I set up a playpen/bassinet right beside my bed. Even though we weren't actually sleeping together, I could hear my baby breathing all night and he could hear me. If my baby cried, whimpered, or gurgled, I could respond immediately. I was very close, but still, my baby was safe, and he was learning to sleep on his own. I transitioned my babies from sleeping in my room to sleeping in their own rooms at around four months old. That's my recipe for baby and Mommy sleeping success.

You will especially appreciate having trained your children to sleep in their own beds as they grow up. My kids learned boundaries and respect for nighttime. People often ask me how I get any sleep with four young children. The truth is, we all get a good night sleep, all night, every night. I never allowed our kids to climb into bed and sleep with us at bedtime. They understood and accepted the rule that they must sleep in their own beds. But I did let them climb into bed with us in the morning, if they wanted. A Saturday morning snuggle is a lovely way to start a weekend together—especially after all kids and parents have had a good night's sleep!

CHAPTER 21

Putting Baby to Sleep

> Why are there dead worms in my bed?
> —Me

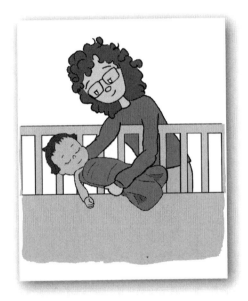

I t is OK to nurse your baby to sleep! Many mothers worry their babies will get too used to it and that could cause a problem later. Don't worry about later right now; worry about now. Now your baby is a newborn, and falling asleep on your breast is completely natural, good, and perfect. You can easily break your baby of this habit later (see chapter 29, "Sleep Training"). For now, it is a perfect way for your baby to fall asleep. You are both relaxed and cozy. When your baby falls asleep and the nipple falls out of her mouth, gently lift her, rest her head on your shoulder, and tap her back for a few minutes to see if she will burp. Kiss your angel,[115] ♪ and then gently lay her down on her back in her crib to sleep. Her arms will spread and her knees will fall outward, legs resembling those of a frog. Note: I never swaddled my babies after we returned home from the hospital. I saw how my babies liked to sprawl out, and I felt that swaddling them restricted them. It's a personal choice. I know some moms whose babies liked to be swaddled. When you lay her down, always rest her bottom down first, then her head. Be sure to place her gently and move slowly so you don't startle her. It's OK, and actually good, if your baby wakes up slightly when you lay her down. She will get to know that her crib is the place for sleeping, which is helpful later when she's more aware of her surroundings. If she's already used to sleeping in her crib, then it's easy to continue to put her to bed there as she grows.

If she wakes up and cries when you lay her down, just talk to her calmly and tell her it's time to sleep. Get her all snug in her sleep bag, and she'll likely stop crying and go to sleep quickly. If you do this right from the get-go, she'll get used to sleeping in her crib. A little cry is just her way of adjusting to the notion of giving in to sleep. If she really starts crying, pick her up and try burping her again; if that doesn't work, try nursing her again, and repeat the above exercise.

Babies need to be put to bed lying on their backs—the safest way for them to sleep. Avoid using blankets, as babies can kick off the blankets and get cold or, worse, the blankets can wiggle up onto the baby's face. You want your baby's face to be free and clear of all items to guarantee unobstructed breathing. Use sleep sacks that fasten with a zipper. These are just like a cozy blanket that your baby wears. They go on over your baby's clothes and zip up to keep him warm and cozy. If you suspect the sleep sack is not warm enough, place a knit blanket

---

115 "Lullabye (Goodnight, My Angel)," Billy Joel, *River of Dreams*, 1993, Columbia Records.

on top of your baby. Be sure to tuck it in snugly so it won't easily come off. You can also fold a small receiving blanket and place it inside the sleep sack to keep your baby warm. If your baby's fingers get cold, put an extra sweater on her at night.

You may find your baby is standing up in her sleep sack, then tripping on it and bumping her head on the crib. She will likely learn to stop doing that pretty quickly, but if she doesn't, then get a sleep sack with legs.[116] Alternatively, pay a seamstress to make a sleep sack with legs out of an existing sleep sack (or sew it yourself—if you can do that, I'm very impressed). I just used what I call "snugglies." I dressed my babies in layers—sweater, cozy vest, and extra jogging pants. This getup worked instead of a blanket. Don't put toys or pillows in the crib with your baby, as these are also suffocation hazards.

Take note of the sleep cry! Sometimes babies have a dream that makes them cry, but they are not awake. It's usually a short burst of crying that stops after a few seconds. You don't need to go to your baby the instant you hear that: wait a few minutes, and she'll likely be quiet again. Additionally, sometimes babies stir and wake slightly in their sleep, but if left undisturbed, they'll quickly fall back asleep. I learned that the hard way after rushing to my baby with every slight sound he made and scooping him up, thinking he needed me to console him. It took a while to realize I was the one waking the baby! Try my rule of thumb if you hear your baby crying in the night: get up and go to the bathroom. Usually by the time you're done, your baby will have quieted down and gone back to sleep. If she's still crying, it's not a sleep cry, so go ahead and soothe or try to troubleshoot the issue, and put her back to bed. Note: tiny newborns need to be tended to right away. Once they are two months old, or so, then put my sleep cry strategy into effect.

I never used traditional bumper pads on my crib because of decreased airflow and an increased risk of SIDS (sudden infant death syndrome). I see the value of bumper pads, as babies can roll and bump their head on the crib rails and can get their chubby little legs and arms stuck between them. Fortunately, the company Safety 1st has invented the perfect solution: an airflow bumper pad. It contains

---

116 Tamara Adamson, teacher and mom

holes and is thin, but can still cushion the blow if a tiny head bumps the rail. I love this product!

When you put your newborn to bed, watch which way her head naturally falls when she's sleeping. If your baby sleeps on both sides of her head equally, that's great. You'll need to pay attention if your baby favors one side of her head for sleeping. My youngest, Maxwell, always slept with his head falling to the right. I was afraid of him getting a flat spot on that side of his head, so I usually gently rolled his head to the left; he stayed that way for the first phase of sleep, then rolled his head the other way at some point. Allowing the skull to rest on both sides helps it to develop into a nice, even shape.

When Baby is sleeping, don't be a control freak about keeping the house quiet. It's OK to play music downstairs and talk in a loud voice, and if you have older kids, it's fine for them to make moderate noise. With some regular household noise, your baby will become a good, solid sleeper who doesn't wake at every sound.

CHAPTER 22

Bathing Baby

What about my stinky ear?
—P., AGE FOUR

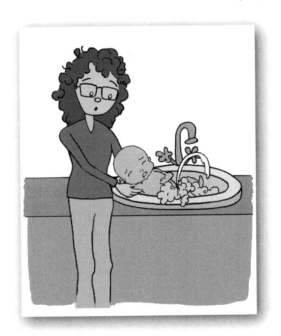

"What is that smell of stinky cheese?"—Mom
"I think that's the baby."—Dad
"What? I just gave her a bath this morning!"—Mom
"Perhaps you missed a spot..."—Dad

Smelly? Crusty? Flaky? Not my baby! Um, yes. No matter how perfect your tiny one is, he will need to have a bath. Splish splash![117] ♪ Bathing a newborn can be a tricky job. First, the baby's head is all floppy, and he can't keep himself in the right position. You need to hold his head to prevent drowning while you wash all the crevices thoroughly. Due to adorable chubbiness, there are a lot of crevices and wrinkles. If you don't get right into these and clean them out, then a stinky cheese smell is likely to appear, along with a thick white film. (If left alone long, it can turn black.) Areas especially prone to film production are under the neck, the armpits, behind the ears, and the folds between the groin and the thighs. It's best to towel-dry these tricky crevices thoroughly after the bath, because air won't naturally reach those spots. You physically have to separate the folds of skin with your finger, wash, and then repeat to dry. Additionally, smearing olive oil or petroleum jelly in these high-risk spots keeps gunk from getting in, preventing the buildup of the stinky cheese stuff. It also protects these spots from becoming red and irritated.

I found that tactic especially important for under the neck. All the folds in the neck and its proximity to dripping milk make it a high-risk spot for irritation. My daughter, Evelyn, had a serious stench coming from behind her ear. I remembered my sister's baby having this problem as well.[118] She ended up calling our local health-care hot line. For both babies, it ended up being a secret crevice of crusty old milk hiding behind the ear. Another parenting dilemma solved!

The belly button needs to be left alone when your baby is fresh from the hospital and it's still long and hasn't fallen off yet. It's OK to bathe your baby, but I never touched the crusty, black skin that was shriveling up. Just keep it dry and clean and don't fiddle with it. Yes, it is gross and it smells (*simply* because it's decaying skin). But leave it alone, and it will fall off. Once your baby is older, and the belly button has healed up and looks like a normal belly button, be sure to start cleaning it during bath

---

117 "Splish Splash," Bobby Darin, *Bobby Darin, 1958,* Atlantic Studios, New York, Atco Records.

118 Ellen Ryan-Chan, teacher and mom

time. Take a cotton swab and gently massage the navel to get any black grimy dirt out. Make sure to be extremely gentle, and don't push the swab into your baby's belly.

If your baby has a flaky, scaly scalp, it is likely cradle cap. Some degree of it is common for infants. It goes away on its own and does not need to be treated. It is ugly and really bugs moms, but it is harmless. No matter how tempting, you are not supposed to pick at cradle cap. I lightly flake off the loose bits of skin with the back of my thumbnail. Then I put a small amount of olive oil or petroleum jelly on my baby's scalp and rub it in. I let it sit for a while and then use a gentle shampoo to remove the loose skin and the oily residue. That is the best way to make your baby's cradle cap look less like snakeskin and more like the head of a perfect little doll.

Many newborns hate being bathed. They scream in terror. Their little eyes are saying, "Mommy! What are you doing to me? Get me out of here!" I have hit on the solution to this problem: water temperature. Parents often make the baby's bathwater too cold. I make my babies' bathwater nice and warm, and they love it because it feels good. Of course, you have to be very careful not to make it too hot; you do not want to burn the baby under any circumstances.

Be sure to use only a little bit baby soap. Too much can cause itching. Rinse with clean water, and, if you like, massage your baby with a gentle, unscented baby lotion.

Special alert: babies are known to pee in the bath. And what is the point in bathing them in pee water? That's slightly counterproductive, isn't it? It's easy to tell when baby boys pee in the bath (did we install a fountain feature in the tub?) but impossible with baby girls. Another reason the rinse at the end is such an important step.

When your baby is confidently sitting up on his own and perhaps interested in grabbing things and moving around, it's time to lose the baby bath. Your baby is ready to splash and explore the big tub! Attention: keep one hand on the baby at *all* times. Do not let go of your baby for even a second. Bathtubs are very slippery, and your baby would not be able to lift himself out of the water to breathe if he slipped. It's a good idea to use a nonslip bathmat and a puffy blow-up cover for the tap (to prevent head-bumping). Get some fun bath toys, and you're good to go.

CHAPTER 23

Fussy Baby

My tummy is hurt, and I have a heck ache.
—E., AGE TWO

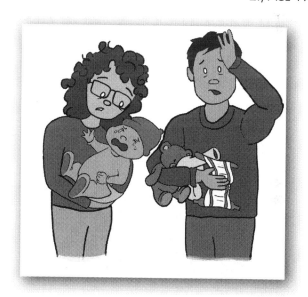

Most babies go through a fussy period each day when they cry and cry for no apparent reason. For my babies, it was always in the late evening, also known as the witching hour. Your baby could be suffering from one of the following: is hungry, is thirsty, has the hiccups, is tired, has a dirty diaper, has a sore bottom, needs to burp, has a tummy ache, is about to spit up or throw up, or has a booger and is annoyed by it. Once all of these possibilities are ruled out, if the baby is still crying, then your baby is having a fussy time.

In my experience, when a baby is behaving like this, she is tired and fighting off sleep.[119] Rock the baby and help her fall asleep. My babies all loved being bounced. Hold the baby upright and rest her head on your shoulder. Hold her close, cuddle her in, gently bounce from your knees and rock from side to side. The movement helped my babies drift off when they were feeling cranky. Once Baby falls asleep, all will be better. In the meantime, here are my notes on the other causes of crying.

Hunger

This one is simple: offer the breast (or bottle if bottle-feeding).

Thirst

Offer the breast (or bottle).

Hiccups

Hiccups really make little babies mad. The best way to get rid of them is to offer the breast (or bottle).

Tired

Offer the breast (or bottle or pacifier). Babies sometimes need a little help getting to sleep when they feel overtired. Often, breastfeeding is the ticket. Some experts say you shouldn't breastfeed to sleep or the baby will become dependent on it. Hogwash! I always breastfed my babies to sleep, and I still successfully sleep trained them all (more on this later). When babies are so tiny and small, they love to breastfeed. It is calming and soothing. What better way to fall into a peaceful, lovely sleep! If baby is tired, breastfeed away.

---

119 Mary Miller, teacher and mom

Grumpy Husband

Offer the breast (sorry, bottle/pacifier is unlikely to work here). Who knew that so many problems could be solved with your breasts? It's pretty impressive, actually; they're almost the solution to everything!

Dirty Diaper

Simple: change the diaper.

Needs White Noise

I have heard that white noise might calm fussy infants. When my first baby, Terrek, had a bad fussy period, my husband or I would run the hair dryer, and the sound did settle him down. I've also heard the hiss of a vaporizer or the midcycle thrum of a washing machine can be successful.

Sore Bottom

Diaper rash can hurt. The best advice I got with respect to preventing it was to always wipe the bottom dry with a tissue after using a wet baby wipe.[120] Staying dry is the best way to avoid the problem. In addition, change your baby often. Don't let her little bottom sit in a dirty diaper. Applying zinc oxide cream also helps some babies. For more information on treating diaper rash, see chapter 19, "Diapering Baby."

Needs Burping

The routine of feeding a newborn includes nursing and burping, nursing and burping, repeat. Burping is a vital part of the picture; those air bubbles can cause discomfort and spit-ups! If a newborn is crying and continues to bring his knees up to his chest, that's a sure sign of gas.[121]

---

120 Charmayne Richards, teacher and mom
121 May Griffin, mom, grandmother, and great grandmother of thirty-six children

There are many different types of burps. There are tiny, soft burps that slip out easily and there are harsh burps that make Baby raise knees to chest and cry in pain. There are wet burps and dry burps, burps that smell like sour milk, burps that turn into little spit-ups, and burps that cause huge vomits where the milk shoots out of Baby's mouth and nose. There are burps that cause mild grimaces and burps that cause sad frowns; there are burps that take two seconds to pop out and Baby doesn't even notice, and there are burps that require endless bouncing and patting until they finally emerge. There are burps that never come, and there are burps that come out in groups. Burps that keep everyone up in the night, burps that sound like a whispering mouse, and burps that sound like a rude old man. Burps, burps, and lots of burps!

Your goal: get the baby to burp after feeding. Your reality: some-times the baby will burp, and sometimes she won't! Try your best with back patting, putting pressure on the tummy, and holding Baby upright so the gas will rise. The most common burping position is resting Baby upright and leaning his head on your shoulder while you pat his back. You can also stand and bounce him; the up-and-down motion helps move the gas. Sometimes the action of lying him down and picking him up again is enough to move the burp up and out. My husband's grand and successful burp-remover maneuver is holding the baby in his arms, one hand under the baby's head and one under the baby's bottom and legs, and gently but briskly folding baby slightly up and down, up and down. It's a useful tactic when Baby is having a very fussy time and the burp just won't cooperate. Putting Baby on her back and rotating her legs like a bike rider also helps move the gas. You want the baby to burp before you lay her down to sleep so that she is less likely to spit up and cry later; however, it doesn't always work out that way. The difficult burping stage won't last forever. As your baby grows, she will soon be able to burp by herself (approximately seven to eight months).

Tummy Ache

My babies were never colicky, so I was lucky that way. From what I hear about colicky babies, they need to move. Rocking, walking, and bouncing (see above) helps to get through the constant crying.[122] Sometimes tummy aches just mean the baby has gas, and the gas has to move up. Try the burping methods discussed above. Sometimes the baby needs to toot. Try putting the baby on her back and rolling her legs in a bicycle motion or pushing her legs up on her abdomen and bringing them down again.[123] You can sing a song to help make her smile.

Spit-Up

Newborn babies spit up a lot. It's always handy to have a receiving blanket or burp cloth over your shoulder when burping your baby to save you from throwing your shirts in the laundry again and again. This frequent spitting up is what gives newborn infants the soft, sweet smell of slightly sour milk. Spit-up will occur less as your baby grows.

Projectile Vomiting

Sometimes spit-ups turn into throw-ups or projectile vomits of such strength the liquid shoots out like a geyser. This was the case with my first and fourth babies. Terrek had huge, powerful vomits often, which freaked me out. I thought something was wrong with him. My pediatrician assured me he was healthy. Some babies just throw up a lot, partly because they drink a lot of milk (perhaps even too much to fit in that tiny tummy). Milk is liquid and churns in the baby's tummy, and sometimes it has no way to escape but through the baby's mouth or nose. (Once, Terrek vomited right into my husband's mouth! He was lying on the couch, holding the baby up for a "fun" helicopter ride at the time.) After witnessing lots of these devastating vomits that soaked my hair, the baby, the rocking chair, the floor, the wall, and me, I began to figure out how to predict them. If you can do that, you can get yourself and your baby off the chair or the carpet and into the bathroom to lean the baby

---

122 Patricia Ryan, teacher and mom

123 http://www.parents.com/baby/care/gas/signs-newborn-has-gas/

over the sink or tub. If you can't make it that far, at least you can aim the baby's mouth at the changing table, making cleanup a lot easier.

The baby is silent before a projectile vomit, almost eerily silent. Additionally, he makes a quiet sound in the back of his throat—like he is clearing it, as if about to make a speech. For the moment right before the baby vomits, he holds his breath so you can't hear his breathing. If you listen closely, sometimes you can hear an odd glub in his belly. These signal that a big vomit is coming, so get prepared. Immediately after a huge vomit like that, the baby is extremely upset and will cry, but shortly after, he realizes that he is hungry again and will need to nurse to refill the tummy he has just emptied, and all is well again.

Projectile vomiting usually ends when the baby starts getting solid foods into his system. Terrek stopped doing it at around six months. Maxwell, on the other hand, continued to eject vomit until he was eleven months old, partly because he did not eat much solid food yet (more on that later!). If you are concerned about your baby's projectile vomits, check with your pediatrician. Note: projectile vomiting will delay sleep training.

Boogers

If you hear your baby snorting, it's likely he has a booger stuck up a nostril, interfering with breathing and making him mad! When I first heard Terrek snort, I got all worried. Did my baby have a snoring problem, asthma, or a respiratory infection? Should I take him to the doctor? I was in a tizzy, and I had my husband go buy a humidifier. A day later, Terrek sneezed out an enormous booger. The snorting immediately ceased. I had no idea an item that large could fit in my baby's tiny nostril. Three babies later, I now have become a master at removing baby's boogers. If you hear your baby snorting, here are some strategies to try.

If you can see the booger, it's a lot easier. Try to pick it out gently with your pinky fingernail. I always kept one pinky fingernail long to make that easier.[124] If you can't quite reach the thing, try squirting the nostril

---

124 Shalimar Santos-Comia, RN and mom

with saline nasal spray. On the other hand, the baby-nose-suction device that comes with baby care kits was useless for me. I just did not have success with that device. What works exceptionally well is sucking the baby's nostril with your own mouth.[125] I know that sounds disgusting, but with your own beautiful baby whom you made with your own flesh and blood, it doesn't seem so gross. Anyway, usually when you suck the nostril, it works to move the booger down far enough that you can reach it; it rarely comes out into your mouth. Alternatively, getting your baby to sneeze can work: take the end of a tissue and touch it gently to your baby's nose just enough to tickle it. Whatever trick you use, it's so gratifying when you finally remove the blockage from your baby's tiny nostrils. The snorting stops, and you both breathe easier.

Temperature

Sometimes the solution to fussiness is as simple as temperature. Is your baby too cold? Too hot? Feel her tiny hands, or touch the back of her neck to assess whether it's hot and sweaty. Maybe you've bundled up your baby too much, maybe not bundled enough. Experiment with layers, and your baby will let you know when she is comfortable.

Remember, the fussy baby stage is short-lived. (Thank goodness!) While it is difficult, draining, and feels like it will never end, it will, and sometimes when you look at your big kid running around and climbing the fence, you will actually miss it! This is the time to remember.[126] ♪

FUSSY BABY CHECKLIST	
☑ Hungry	☑ Temperature
☑ Thirsty	☑ Diaper change
☑ Boogers/stuffy nose	☑ Gas (burp, toot)
☑ Hiccups	☑ Spit-up/vomiting
☑ Tummy ache	☑ Tired

---

125 Ibid.

126 "This Is the Time," Billy Joel, *The Bridge*, 1986, Columbia Records.

CHAPTER 24

Sick Baby

> Mommy, I have a tummy ache in my throat.
> —E., AGE TWO

When your baby gets sick for the first time, it's tempting to panic. The first time Terrek had a fever, my husband and I took him to the hospital emergency room. (Talk about freaking out for no reason!) He was fine; he just needed some baby fever medication. Here's some news: your baby will get sick, and then your baby will get better. That is how it works. It's actually good for your baby to get sick, so don't be too paranoid about germs; they can strengthen his immune system in the long run.[127] It is bothersome and exhausting when your tiny infant has a cold, but after four tiny infants going through it, I have come up with a few tips to make it less painful for everyone involved.

The first thing I always do if I notice my infant is getting a runny nose is try to get the same cold. (If bottle feeding; no need to do this). I deliberately expose myself to my little baby's germs—and this, my friend, is very easy to do. There is snot and slobber everywhere, believe me. If your body, with a well-established immune system, is fighting the same virus, it will be much easier on your baby. When you breastfeed, your body is providing your baby with antibodies to fight the bad germs. You are acting as an immune system for your baby.

---

127 http://www.webmd.com/parenting/d2n-stopping-germs-12/kids-and-dirt-germs

This is the best thing you can do to help your baby get well soon. Yes, it sucks because it means you have to get a cold. You're already sleep deprived, and you still have to exert all your energy to care for your baby (and possibly other kids), but if you are acting in your new baby's best interests, this is the sacrifice you make.

Next, I give my baby an over-the-counter homeopathic remedy also said to help fight colds—a clear liquid called Coreazalia. Although I have not performed clinical studies on its effectiveness, when I have used Coreazalia, the cold seemed neither as severe nor to last as long as usual (without any form of treatment).

Life is very difficult for a baby when she has a stuffy nose. Very young infants don't yet know how to breathe through their mouths, so they depend on their noses for air. Nursing also requires nose breathing, and when your stuffed-up baby has to stop nursing to gasp for air through his mouth, he is not a happy camper.

For relief, I try pediatric saline nasal spray. My method: squirt it in one nostril and then suck it out with my mouth, to loosen things up inside the nostril and draw out fluid. You'll need a cloth to spit in after this. Then I repeat the process on the other side. I understand this sounds completely gross, but believe me, when your innocent little baby is hungry, sick, tired, and struggling to breathe, you'll do anything. And this tactic actually helps. Your baby will hate the process and will sputter and cough, gag, cry loudly, and act like he's drowning, but, soon after, he'll be able to breathe through his nose effectively enough to nurse and then fall asleep—a huge relief. Milk and sleep will make him recover.

A vaporizer or humidifier in the baby's room can also help him feel better. Moist air feels gentler to breathe when you have a sore throat. Be sure to let the room dry out thoroughly later so you don't encourage mold to grow, and take care not to let water sit in the machine; I know from experience that a clear slime can develop. Thoroughly dry the humidifier or vaporizer, after it has been running all night, each morning. Take it apart, empty it, and place it over a vent or near a fan. Although the instruction manuals always recommend regular cleaning with bleach, I refuse to use such a harsh and toxic chemical in a device that directly influences the air my baby breathes.

Another tip for unblocking sinuses: bring your baby into the bathroom and let her rest in the bouncy chair during your shower. The hot steam will go to work on her nasal passages so she can breathe better.

I can always tell right away if my baby has a fever. You get used to the natural warm feel of your baby, and when her temperature is rising, you can easily detect it, especially when you're cheek-to-cheek. The baby's skin will feel hot. A digital ear thermometer can verify the hunch with just one push of a button. If her temperature is higher than normal (36°C or 98.6°F), give her fever medication.

Since babies hate medicine even more than cats do, this won't be easy. Medicine has a strong sugary flavor, and there is a lot of it to get into Baby's mouth. Infant fever medication comes with a syringe; use it instead of a spoon. Only squirt in a little bit at a time, as babies don't know how to swallow a lot of liquid at once. If you squirt too much, he'll sputter, cough, choke, and gag, and he may throw up (eliminating all the medicine you just administered). I always buy the dye-free baby fever medication that lasts for eight hours (read labels). It lasts for the entire night, and I like that it is clear with no added food colors.

Additionally, wipe a feverish baby down with a cool, wet cloth. Dress her in light pajamas and use a light sleep sack or none at all.

The best advice for caring for a sick baby is lots of cuddling. Snuggle up in the rocking chair and rest there while your baby rests, too. You'll get through this together and be that much stronger.

CHAPTER 25

Baby Sign Language

> I found where the worms are coming
> from—from the boys' pockets.
> —ME

Using sign language with your baby is an exciting way to establish communication well before he is able to speak. With all my children, I found it a helpful, special way to connect. It reduces some of the frustrated crying that babies do when they can't get their messages across and makes it easier to figure out what your baby wants. Babies feel a sense of pride when they sign and know they've been understood.

I always spoke with my babies as if they *could* understand. I would explain things to them that some might think were way beyond the babies' ability to comprehend—and perhaps they were, but, on the other hand, this type of rich dialogue may have contributed to my children's advanced language skills. Who knows? While I spoke with them, I would always sign. If they screamed at me, I would calmly say, "Don't scream. Use your sign." My babies eventually got this, and our wonderful back-and-forth flourished.

Some people believe baby sign language might act as a crutch to delay actual speaking. That didn't happen to my children: all were early speakers and developed a large and fluid vocabulary before age two. When I did my education master's thesis, I learned that movement and actions can actually facilitate learning,[128] and I believe this to be the case with sign language for babies. On the other hand, if your child does happen to be speech delayed, knowing sign language could greatly help facilitate communication.

I didn't go crazy teaching my babies the entire dictionary, just a few choice signs that were key in their schema of life. I taught them *milk, more, done, change, eat, drink, sorry, thank-you,* and *please*. My babies and I also figured out our own additional signals for *where, up, yes, no, shhh,* and *don't touch*. Teaching your baby such signs is easier than you might think.

I started when they were around four months old. I know babies cannot contribute to the conversation at that age; I was trying to get a jump on training myself, and I hoped the baby would begin to connect the action with the spoken word right from the get-go. I'm not sure when they actually started doing that, but I believe that babies can understand a lot more than people give them credit for. It is truly a thrill when your tiny baby starts to sign back, and you know you've made a real connection.

Whenever I said certain phrases to the baby, like, "Do you want milk?" or, "It's time for milk," I would always sign the word for *milk* close enough so that my baby could see. If it was time to change the diaper I would say, "change" and make the sign for *change* as I began. Using these simple signs along with the words came very naturally after a while.

Teaching *more* and *done* is the easiest; these will likely be the first two signs your baby masters. At six months, as you start feeding your baby solid foods, say the words *more* and *done* frequently during the meal, and make the signs for each as you say each word. Soon, these signs are easily transferable to nonfood situations. For example, *done*, as in "I'm *done* with the boat, Mommy. I want out! *Done*." Or "*more* horsey ride Grandpa, *more!*" When feeding, you can also introduce *eat* and *drink*. "Are you hungry?" "Do you want to *eat?*" "Do you

---

128 Ryan, Charlotte *Creative Movement: A Powerful Strategy to Teach Science.* 2006. Toronto, ON: University of Toronto

want a *drink* of water?" Speak to your baby a lot and sign with these familiar words *every time* you say them. Your baby will pick them up.

Babies' signs may not look exactly like the signs are technically supposed to. Terrek's *more* sign had one finger pointing to the other palm, and for a while, Maxwell's *more* sign was his two index fingers tapping each other. This doesn't matter. As long as you get your baby's point and you're communicating, then you are successful.

You might be surprised how the regular gestures you already make are perfect signs for your baby. Around the twelve-month mark, these can work their way into your baby's sign language vocabulary. For instance, for *where, yes, no, up, shhh, hi,* and *bye,* I did not use the American Sign Language sign. It came naturally to use body language instead—shaking and nodding our heads for *yes* and *no,* and extending hands with elbows bent for *where,* as if wondering where something was. For *up,* as in "I want up; pick me up!" my baby just raised his arms toward me, and my automatic response was to pick him up. Communication was clear. For *shhh,* we used the traditional finger to the lips. It's so cute to watch a little one-year-old telling his big brothers to "shhh." Maxwell also caught on to "no-no-no." When I would shake my pointer finger and mean "no, don't touch," he quickly started doing that when facing something he knew he wasn't allowed to touch. *Hi* and *bye* were, of course, just waving. Once a baby masters *yes* and *no,* communication gets exponentially easier! You can ask a question, and she can answer, long before she is able to speak.

Babies may invent their own signs. Follow their leads, and encourage them to repeat a signal that showed what they wanted. For instance, Maxwell made up his own sign for *want* that stuck. He transitioned from screeching at the top of his lungs and grabbing for things (thank goodness—very embarrassing in public) to putting his hands up and rotating them with fingers spread. It was his way of saying "I want that," and I quickly caught on. I started mirroring this sign when I said the word "want" to reinforce the meaning. He knew what I meant, and I knew what he meant.

The manners signs were the last ones I introduced: after twelve months, I started gently encouraging my babies to say "please" when asking for something, then took their hand and made a *please* sign (American Sign Language). It took them a month or so, but they all caught on and eventually did it themselves. I did the same with *thank you*. And if they hit, poked, or scratched, I looked at them, explained that what they did hurt and that they needed to say *sorry*, and again gently moved their hands in the *sorry* gesture. Babies are capable of learning their manners before they can actually verbalize them.

The signs, gestures, and actions you develop with your baby become your own special vocabulary that will help make life together run more smoothly, and with fewer frustrations. Words cannot express how incredibly rewarding baby sign language can be. There should be a sign for that!

As soon as babies begin speaking in audible words, they naturally drop the sign language and it becomes a distant memory. It's helpful for a short time in the baby's life, but it is extremely helpful! Numerous books have been written about baby sign language, and although I didn't read any (I heard about the practice from other moms[129]), here's a link to some reviews: http://www.start-american-sign-language.com/baby-sign-language-books.html.

---

129 Shalimar Santos-Comia, RN and mom

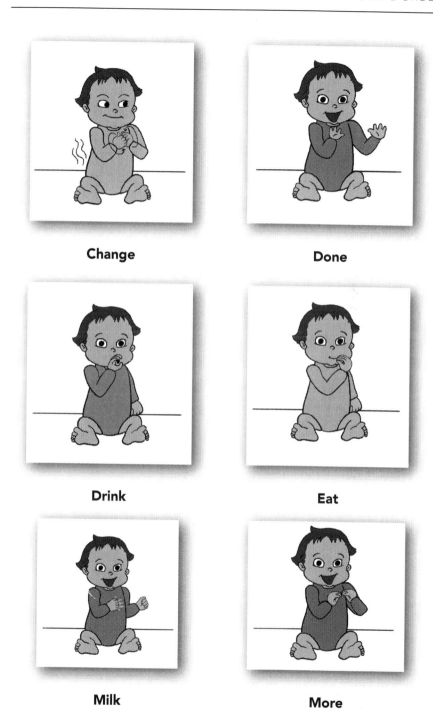

Change

Done

Drink

Eat

Milk

More

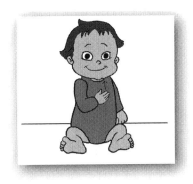

Please

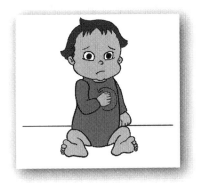

Sorry

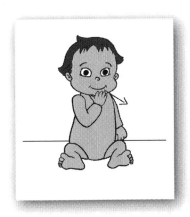

Thank you

CHAPTER 26

Making Strange

> Me no like dresses. Bad pretty.
> —E., AGE TWO

"**M**aking strange" refers to when babies are scared and cry when held by someone other than Mom or Dad. Most babies go through a period when they make strange with anyone (or almost anyone). They may be fine with people they see more often, like grandparents. My babies all made strange for a while. It started somewhere late in the fourth month and lasted for many months. This is a completely normal stage in Baby's development.

Think about it from the baby's perspective. He is a completely vulnerable and dependent individual at this time in his life. He has learned that Mommy is his lifeline. Mommy gives him milk; Mommy cuddles him and keeps him safe. Mommy stops the bad burp from hurting him, and Mommy prevents big siblings from poking him in the eye. He has realized that he needs Mommy to survive. If Mommy is suddenly gone, and some stranger is holding him (it could be good old Aunt Edna, but still a stranger to him), his whole world may fall apart. He is thinking, "What if this person drops me? What if this person doesn't feed me? What if Mommy never comes back?"

It's a scary thing for a little baby. So be compassionate. If my baby is afraid of someone holding him, and he is crying, then I'm going to get him back and reassure him that it's OK and that he's safe. Then we both feel better. When crazy Aunt Edna whisks the screaming baby away, trying to "teach" the baby not to make strange (believe me, this will happen), it actually makes things worse. The baby begins to panic more the farther Aunt Edna takes him away from Mommy. The baby will now freak out, believing his worst fear is coming true ("I've been abducted. I can't find Mommy!"). He will just cry harder. The baby is not going to learn not to make strange this way. The baby needs to go through that natural phase of his development knowing his lifeline, his mommy, is there.

You can try a particular strategy to lessen the problem, though it's not necessary and may or may not succeed; nothing is as good as Mommy to the baby right now. If you want to give it a shot, then when good old Aunt Edna holds the baby, stay near, and reassure the baby that it's OK and that you trust Aunt Edna. You need to kiss Aunt Edna and pat her arm, showing Baby that you know Aunt Edna is holding him and that it's safe. If Aunt Edna starts walking away and Baby starts screaming, Aunt Edna should say, "It's OK, Baby. Do you want your mommy? I will take you to your mommy." Then Aunt Edna needs, actually, to take the baby to mommy.[130]

If Baby sees Aunt Edna regularly, and Aunt Edna doesn't deny Baby his mommy, then the baby will learn to trust Aunt Edna and will stop making strange. If Baby only sees Aunt Edna at Christmas and the odd birthday, then Baby will likely not stop making strange with her. Whisking Baby away while he is screaming is not helping anyone. It's just scaring and traumatizing the poor little baby! Give Baby back to his mommy, you meanie!

---

130 Patricia Ryan, teacher and mom

CHAPTER 27

Teething and Caring for Baby Teeth

Mommy, I love you more than a crab.

—P., Age Three

Before your baby actually starts growing teeth, she will start drooling, a lot! (This happened at around three months of age for my babies.) It's time to pull out the "drool bibs." The purpose of these is to keep the cute outfit underneath the bib dry. You'll need a lot, as they become soaking wet quickly. I prefer small ones without the crinkly plastic backing. Additionally, the kind that snap at the side of the neck are so much easier to put on and take off than all the other varieties.

When your baby starts teething, he will want to chew on everything. That includes everything he can get his hands on. The baby will pick something up, and it will go immediately into his mouth. Babies will even want to chew on you (arm, shoulder, finger, chin, nipple!). Ouch—babies can bite. (Hello, Maxwell!) Try providing cold, wet washcloths to chew on and baby chew-toys. I like the variety filled with water that chills in the fridge.

Some babies breeze through this period with minimal concern (my first three). However, some babies have a lot of trouble with teething (Maxwell—you again!). If this is the case for your little one, you may want to do something to help him through this difficult time. I avoided over-the-counter oral gel; it can numb the mouth and make nursing harder.[131] Instead, try infant fever medication for the pain. A homeopathic teething product by Boiron called Camilia may also help. I didn't have to use medication or remedies very often, but they did help a few times.

Babies may also develop a low fever from teething. My first son, Terrek, did. My husband and I were on vacation with him at the time, and we panicked, bringing him to the local emergency room. The doctor looked at him, informed us he was teething, and recommended medication.

A teething baby can get a red rash on his face from all the drool. Try to keep his face dry. Apply a thin layer of petroleum jelly if the skin is irritated. Soon your baby will have little tiny teeth! It looks so funny at first, but you'll quickly get used to his new little smile.

I recall seeing a poster from the health department once—it showed a photo of a baby going to bed in his crib while sucking on a lollypop. The poster conveyed the message that, in terms of sugar and tooth decay, this wasn't any different from letting your baby fall asleep while drinking milk. That convinced me I had to do something to protect my baby's clean new teeth without giving up the special comfort of nursing him to dreamland. By wiping your baby's teeth, you can have it all. Your baby will eventually get used to it and realize, "It's just Mommy taking good care of me again."

It *is* important to take care of your baby's teeth. While it's too early for a toothbrush and toothpaste, giving drinks of water after feeding can help rinse away any food residue. I always wiped my baby's teeth with a wet cloth after nursing or feeding[132] to wipe away sugars and prevent tooth decay, even during the night. "What? Are you crazy, wake a sleeping baby to wipe their teeth? You'd have to be a fool to do such a thing!" is what you may be thinking. Well, true, the baby will most likely wake up ticked off. That's OK. It's a bit of a nuisance at the beginning, but once he gets used to the teeth-wiping routine, he will be only mildly irritated and drift right back to sleep. One silver

---

131 Mary Miller, teacher and mom

132 http://www.aboutkidshealth.ca/En/HealthAZ/HealthandWellness/DentalCare/Pages/Teeth-Dental-Care.aspx

lining: this is early training for learning to get back to sleep in a crib on his own.

If it's particularly hard for your baby to settle after teeth-wiping, be proactive. Have your damp cloth ready and wipe her teeth while she is still in your arms. Then you can gently rock her back to sleep before you place her in the crib. You might find it helpful to whisper a little explanation as you wipe so the baby learns what to expect: "Teeth time. I'm just cleaning your little teeth," and then, "Done! I'm done." My babies knew the word *done* by then, from signing at feeding time. When they heard *done*, they would settle down and go back to sleep.

Around eleven to twelve months, I introduced a baby toothbrush (it looks like a little finger glove with some bristles on it) and infant toothpaste (fluoride-free—safe for swallowing). Warning: babies will bite your finger! Be prepared; their jaws are very strong. Soon, after the baby is twelve months old, you can switch to a soft toddler tooth-brush. Keep using the infant toothpaste until age three, and transition to a regular kids' toothpaste with fluoride, as he'll now be able to spit it out without swallowing the chemicals. Keep those pearly whites in tiptop shape, so that in a few years your child can leave lovely, healthy teeth for the Tooth Fairy!

CHAPTER 28

Solid Foods

It's a good thing the squash exploded.
—P., Age Four

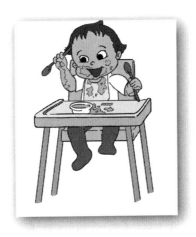

ntroducing solid foods is such an exciting step in your baby's life. I always videotaped the first few introductions of mush that inevitably cause cute frowns and adorable grimaces. Warning: most babies appear to hate solid foods at first. Babies go through an adjustment period when they need to get used to new textures and different tastes, and it all seems completely strange and foreign to them. Although Baby may dodge the spoon by turning her head or holding her mouth shut tight when the spoon approaches, don't give up. While you should never force your baby to eat, keep trying with different foods, even if you can only get her to taste a tiny little bit. Be happy. Show your baby that eating is fun. Open your mouth wide to show your baby how it is done. Eventually your baby should develop tastes for food, will relish it, and will ask for more. This was true with my first three, who hated baby food at the beginning until they grew to like it. My fourth, little Maxwell, was a different story…more on that later.

All babies have different taste preferences. Terrek loved applesauce; Evelyn hated applesauce but loved green beans. Green beans made Patrick angry, but he loved orange vegetables like yams or squash. Evelyn and Max hated squash. It made them shudder and grimace. If your child seems relentlessly to hate one food, stop offering it for a while. When you reintroduce it later, she will probably like it, unless she's like Maxwell.

Babies have tiny tummies. Start feeding with only tiny amounts of food, and never make your baby eat more than she wants to. When she is done, she is done! This is an excellent time to work on the sign language words for *done* and *more*. Your baby will pick them up quickly. Remember breast milk or formula is still your baby's main staple for nourishment right now.

Here is the feeding program I used with my babies: at six months old, I always started with rice cereal mixed with a little bit of breast milk. Remember, a very tiny bit—one teaspoon. I also let my babies begin sipping water at six months. Your baby may sputter and choke at first until he learns to sip and swallow successfully from a cup. He will think this sipping water business is great fun! He soon will fight to put his hands in it. Babies also love water in a baby bottle, a preface to drinking milk from it in the future. Practicing with water is a great way to get them to learn how to use a bottle. I don't bother with juices because they have high sugar content, unless it's freshly squeezed (try carrot-apple—babies love this). I introduce oat cereal next. I then try vegetable purees, then fruits. Around eight months, I start adding tofu, lentils, scrambled eggs, chicken, turkey, and fish into the mix as well as other grains. I also offer rice husks to chew on at this age and other soft foods to explore. I introduce dairy by eleven months (cheese and yogurt). At twelve months, my babies no longer want the mushy stuff and are ready to nibble on "real" food.

A note about sensitivities: be sure to introduce only one food at a time so you can watch for any allergic reactions. When my first three babies were little, medical experts were advising parents to wait until certain ages before introducing potentially allergic foods— twelve months for dairy and eggs, eighteen months for shellfish, and three years for nuts (a major choking hazard). However, by the time baby Maxwell came around, that advice had changed. The Canadian Pediatric Society now recommends trying out such foods with infants as early as six months, positioning that early exposure could help protect against developing an allergy to these foods.[133] When Maxwell was six months old, I dipped my finger in a tiny bit of peanut butter and put it in his mouth. I also let him try scrambled eggs and a touch of fish and shrimp when he was only seven months old. Do not feed babies honey: it poses a risk of botulism, which could make your baby very sick.[134]

Making your own baby food is actually not that difficult. Just steam the veggies and puree in a blender or food processor. Freezing the baby food in ice cube trays[135] creates perfectly sized portions that are always fresh. As your baby gets old enough for a larger variety of foods, you can blend up for his meal some of whatever you are having for dinner.

Some babies enjoy munching on actual solid pieces of food from a very young age.[136] Sucking on part of a broccoli or a plum can be very satisfying and can aid in the transition from baby food to grown-up food. If your baby grabs for your food while you are eating, let him try it (as long as it is healthy with no added salt or sugar). This is the beginning of a long journey of your child's eating from your plate and vice versa!

---

133 Canadian Pediatric Society, http://www.cps.ca/media/release-communique/no-need-to-delay-introduction-of-food-allergens-to-high-risk-babies, 03/20/2014

134 http://www.babycenter.ca/x555838/is-it-safe-to-give-my-baby-honey, 06/30/2014.

135 Patricia Ryan, teacher and mom

136 Ellen Ryan-Chan, teacher and mom

Unlike my other three babies, Maxwell never grew to like purees. He would purse his lips closed when the spoon approached, and he refused to open his mouth. Some moms find homemade baby food tastes better, and that babies who resisted jarred purees did better with made-from-scratch.[137] Not Maxwell. For him, no mush was good mush! I didn't worry about it too much. Instead of feeding him baby food from a spoon, I would spread it on a rice cake or a rice husk cracker. He would eat it that way on his own. I also let him have simple soft foods that were mostly salt- and sugar-free: steamed veggies, raw cucumber and avocado, fruit, noodles, plain ground chicken, tofu, scrambled eggs, and cereal (oat circles or wheat squares). If your baby is like Maxwell, you may want to read the book *Baby-Led Weaning* for more about this approach.[138] While I didn't adhere to it completely, the book has excellent points and helpful advice. Eventually, I gave up on the purees and just let Maxwell eat real food, plus small servings of baby cereal, which are fortified with iron that's important for a baby's nutrition.

As soon as my babies could hold a spoon, I always let them feed themselves. People were always impressed that my tiny toddlers could feed themselves quite independently. Of course, this is a very messy endeavor at first. The baby will cover herself in food; she will need a bath and a change of clothes, and the table, wall, floor, and high chair will practically need hosing down. But self-feeding pays off. It fosters self-reliance, gives little ones a sense of control, and develops hand-eye coordination. Training your baby to feed himself early gives you some freedom. You won't have to constantly hover and spoon-feed. Eventually, you'll be able to sit down and enjoy your meal while your baby enjoys his.

I avoid junk food for as long as possible—until my baby is old enough to feel the sense of injustice when the older siblings are enjoying a junk food treat. Until then, it's no sugary or salty snacks. Why subject your baby's tiny body to chemicals and food that is not actually

---

137 Tamara Adamson, teacher and mom
138 Gill Rapley and Tracey Murkett, *Baby-Led Weaning* (London: Vermilion, 2008).

going to help her thrive and grow, especially when she doesn't know the difference?

Healthy and yummy toddler snacks include chopped fruit (bananas, blueberries, apples, sliced oranges, plums, peaches, cut-up grapes, pears, cantaloupe, watermelon, papaya, and mango), veggies (cucumber, green beans, peas, corn, celery, broccoli, slightly steamed carrots, and avocado), whole-grain crackers, rice cakes, toast strips, rice husks, dry cereal, raisins, applesauce, cold noodles, cheese, yogurt, edamame, chicken meatballs, hard-boiled eggs, and sunflower seed butter (sold as SunButter). Peanut and other nut and seed butters are healthy and easy options, too, if allergies are not a problem. It's a great idea to get your toddler used to the flavor of SunButter now, since it does not contain nuts, and it's made in a nut-free facility and therefore not problematic to bring to school. When your child goes to school in a few short years, you can send her off with a sandwich of SunButter and jam, which my kids love. Traditional peanut butter and jelly kids' bag lunches are becoming a thing of the past, as many schools today forbid them on campus due to life-threatening allergies (in North America, anyway).

With a change in food comes a change in poo, effective immediately (or as soon as solid foods get into Baby's system). Say good-bye to the mustard poos and hello to a wide assortment and variety of textures, consistencies, colors, and smells. It's a surprise each time! Don't be alarmed if your baby gets backed up and doesn't "go" for the first few days after getting some solid food in her little system. At first, the new presence of solid foods takes a few days to work its way through. If you worry that your baby is constipated, feed her some strained prune baby food; strained pears work, too. Give your baby water in a sippy cup or bottle to help move things along. If she still has difficulty with bowel movements, see your pediatrician.

CHAPTER 29

Sleep Training

Mommy, can you tuck me up?
—P., Age Three

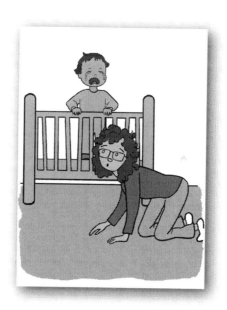

Sleep training is essential for you and your baby. Sleep training means teaching your baby to sleep through the night. She will establish healthy sleep habits to carry with her for the rest of her life, and you can finally rest easy and sleep for eight uninterrupted hours! It's a beautiful thing...once it's accomplished.

The actual week or so of sleep training is hellish and heartbreaking. It's a few hard days' nights.[139] ♪ I'm not going to lie, but after four children, I see that it is the right thing to do. Babies *can* learn to sleep on their own, and—in so doing—they learn boundaries and respect for their parents. Parents who don't sleep train often end up with babies and toddlers who wake in the night for years to come and depend on a parent to help them get to sleep and stay asleep. Interrupted sleep and poor sleep habits are bad for the child and for the parent. So as difficult as this period is, the effort is worth it in the long run.

All my children slept through the night regularly as soon as sleep training was completed. It only takes about one week. The baby won't remember the trauma and angst of wondering why Mommy isn't picking him up, but he will have developed healthy habits for life.

When I was a new mother of just one, I was completely against the idea of letting the baby "cry it out." I never let my baby cry. I let him fall asleep with me, in my bed, and I rocked him, cradled him, and helped him fall asleep. I sang "Frère Jacques" a million times while rubbing his belly. I was so sick of that song! I ended up with a baby who would never sleep on his own. He was completely dependent on me. I spent so much time getting him to fall asleep that I was neglecting my own sleep. I was totally exhausted, burned out, irritable, and cranky, and my husband and I kept getting into arguments. It was a rough time, but looking back, I think it was so rough because I was seriously sleep deprived. My doctor said to me, "You won't let your baby cry, yet you are the one who is crying." Those words stuck with me, and I knew something had to change.

After four children, I have learned two important things about sleep training. The first is that a little bit of crying while the baby is falling asleep is OK. They just need to work through it to get to sleep. They learn to put themselves to sleep. The other is that if you, the mother, are well rested, you can do a much better job of taking care of your kids.

---

139 "Hard Day's Night," The Beatles, *Hard Day's Night*, 1964, EMI Studios, London, Label: Parlophone.

When babies are very little is *not* a time for this training. At that age (under nine months), when they're obviously tired and you lay them down, sometimes just leaving them be for a minute or two is enough for them to drift off on their own. I found that when you have other children and need to run off for a second to help them with the potty, kiss a hurt knee, wipe up spilled milk, and so forth, it gives the baby enough time to fall asleep on his own.

I officially sleep train when my babies are nine months old and never before. I always breastfeed on demand, and when they have such tiny tummies, I feel they need those night feedings. By nine months, they have been on solid foods for three months; additionally, by nine months, your baby is big enough that he can burp by himself, without needing picking up to help ease gas pain. Nine months is still young enough that your baby can adapt quickly, but old enough that he won't automatically need feeding again during the night. You will notice that at nine months, sometimes babies cry out of want, not just need. They are beginning to express their emotions and sometimes just don't want to go to bed. It's time to teach them firmly but lovingly that it is bedtime, and we go to sleep at bedtime. I find that after nine months, imparting that lesson gets harder. Your baby is older and more used to the way things have been. Trying to introduce a major change, such as changing sleep patterns, could take longer if you wait to do so much past this age.

The key to successful sleep training is conviction. When you make up your mind to do it, you must stick to it and not waver. If you end up giving in to your baby's plaintive cries (and believe me they are so pathetic and desperate—babies know how to pull on your heartstrings) it will be even harder to sleep train them going forward. You can't go back. My system is simple, but it requires willpower. For me, when my baby cries, I instinctively want to solve the problem and comfort him. Mommy always makes things better. Sleep training is one of the first times you transfer some ownership to the baby as an individual. Babies learn that they can do something independently, without Mommy, and that something is falling asleep.

As a mom, it's easy to give every part of yourself to your baby. You give him your love, time, energy, attention, and nutrients. If you give him so much that you are not taking care of yourself, that isn't the best thing for the baby. Mom and Baby need to learn that Mom's rest and well-being are important, too. A *good* night's sleep is *good*. You need to get it!

How it works: Make sure your baby is well fed, clean, changed, and comfortable—not too hot, not too cold. Play gentle classical music in the hallway. Lay your baby down in the crib at bedtime, after nursing (and wiping her teeth). Say to your baby, "I love you. It's time for you to sleep now. Nighttime is for sleeping. You are going to sleep all night tonight; I'm so proud of you. I love you, good night." Pat your baby on the tummy, blow her a kiss, then leave. Your baby will most likely cry. Wait for one minute. Go back and lay her back down if she is sitting up or standing, but *do not* pick her up.[140] Simply put your hand on her and say, "I love you. Nighttime is for sleeping." I used a firm but calm voice, so the baby knew I was serious and that everything was OK. You can repeat this statement a few times, or say, "There, there." Then leave the room. Do not linger.

He will know you are nearby; your tone has reassured him that he is safe and not abandoned. Your baby will probably cry again. Wait two minutes. Go back in, and repeat the same process (lay the baby down if he is sitting up, say, "I love you; nighttime is for sleeping," and leave). Baby will cry. Go back in after four minutes and repeat. *Do not pick up the baby.* Then increase the increments to eight minutes, then sixteen minutes. Keep increasing the length of time between visits until the baby falls asleep.

After the baby has been completely quiet for a while, sneak in and check on her. Sometimes she might have her head right up against the crib rails, which could be uncomfortable and wake her. Gently move her; she likely won't wake. A few times, I found Maxwell asleep sitting up, with his face resting against the crib rails. I gently laid him down, and he stayed asleep.

Repeat the same pattern each time your baby wakes for the rest of the night. You can even replay your classical music again. This works as a signal that it's time for sleeping.

---

140 Brenda Cuthbertson, mom

Warning: there will be lots of fussing, screaming, and sobbing. Your baby is wondering, "What is going on? You are always at my beck and call! I'm becking, and I'm calling. Why aren't you helping me? I'm so mad!" Your heart will be breaking, because it's so hard to resist comforting your baby. You will feel like a terrible mother (or father), and you'll want to quit. *Don't!* This won't last much longer. Repeat the same pattern the second night. You'll find that your baby will give up earlier, and you may not even reach the full sixteen minutes. When Baby starts to settle down, and you hear his cries stopping, don't go back in. If you do, you will get him all riled up again, and his crying will get stronger. Just wait patiently outside of his room; he is about to fall asleep. After about a week, your baby will have learned that nighttime is for sleeping, and he won't bother waking up in the night anymore. He won't fuss when you put him to bed. The baby will simply accept it and go to sleep. It sounds too good to be true, but the method works, and you both will be well rested and happy!

I always expected my babies to give me an eight-hour sleep when they were sleep trained. They can sleep much longer than that if you give them a "dream feed." I put my babies to bed at eight o'clock, and then right before I went to bed at ten o'clock or so, I sneaked back into their rooms, gingerly lifted them, and nursed. They usually didn't wake; they'd feed in their sleep. They might have stirred a bit, especially when I wiped their teeth with a cloth (a precursor to brushing, which removes sugars left by the milk and prevents tooth decay). Even if they do wake slightly, just say, "Good night. Nighttime is for sleeping," and they'll drift right back off to sleep. The dream feed keeps them full and helps them last the night. I wouldn't let my babies get up until six o'clock in the morning. If they woke up earlier wanting to nurse, I acted as if it were still night, and they learned when it was OK to wake.

In the morning, give your baby huge hugs and praise! Let her know you are proud of her and so happy she slept all night. Even though she can't talk to you yet, talk to her. She will get the gist of what you are saying. "Good job! You slept through the night. Don't you feel well rested and healthy today? I love you, and I'm so proud of you! Well done!"

Note: sleep training also will eliminate those periods in the night when your baby is wide-awake, giggling at you, and grabbing your nose, and you are thinking, "It's a good thing you're so damn adorable because it's four-thirty in the morning, and I have to get up with your brothers and sister soon!"

Treat nap times the same as nighttime during sleep training. At nine months, your baby will be having a morning and an afternoon snooze. Use the method. Remember, consistency is the key.

Of course, you'll have a setback in sleep training if your baby gets sick. If he has a fever, he will need care and fever medication throughout the night, so you shouldn't let him cry through that. Take care of your baby; you may have to retrain him when he's well again, but it will be much faster and easier this time.

Such is the recipe for sleep training your baby. It's that simple. Sleep! Glorious sleep. It's so *wondrous* to finally have a good night's sleep. Now you and your child will enjoy this healthy and beneficial ritual for years to come!

Note: Don't try to sleep train while your baby wears cloth diapers at night. (When he wets, he will feel cold and soggy. Who could sleep comfortably through that?) I learned that the hard way when I tried to sleep train my first son, Terrek. After recognizing the simple cause of his distress, I felt so bad that I had inadvertently caused it! Don't do it! Use a disposable diaper at night; it makes the baby's bottom feel dry so he can rest.

Finally, if your baby still has problems with projectile vomiting, I suggest waiting until he outgrows that before attempting sleep training. My first son, Terrek, was a projectile vomiter (see Spit-Up in chapter 23, "Fussy Baby,"), but he had long outgrown it by nine months, so he was ready for sleep training. My fourth baby, little Maxwell, on the other hand, was still occasionally projectile vomiting at that age, and I realized sleep training him just wasn't going to happen yet; when I tried, he cried so hard it activated his gag reflex profusely. Of course, when that happens, you must comfort him, bathe him, change him, change the bed, and feed him again. That poses a *slight* problem for sleep training, to say the least. If your baby is like Terrek or Maxwell and eats more than the tummy can hold, or if your baby has a sensitive gag reflex, by all means, wait until he outgrows the projectile phase before you implement the sleep training plan. Sorry—a good night's sleep is still a little further away. Upside: you can cherish rocking and nursing your baby in the night a little longer.

I finally sleep trained Maxwell at eleven months—and did find, as stated earlier, that the older the baby is, the longer it takes. It took approximately two-and-a-half weeks. One last tidbit—if your baby has a bowel movement in the night (rare for nine months old), it goes without saying that you must change him. Never leave a baby in a soiled diaper. With those limitations and notes in mind, good luck to you and your baby! Sleep training works. You will both be relieved and happy when it's over. Enjoy your zzz's! ☺

CHAPTER 30

Babyproofing Your House

Ah! Maxwell coughed up a sticker!

—Me

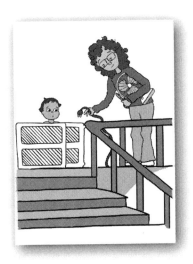

Your baby will likely start crawling at around seven to ten months, so you'll need to babyproof your house before then. This step is essential to ensure the safety of your baby, and it makes your life easier so you don't have to constantly chase after him. (Who am I kidding? No matter what you do, you're always going to be doing that!) No matter how much babyproofing you do (or chasing, for that matter), it's never enough. Babies always manage to get into stuff anyway, freak you out, make a mess, get hurt, and eat something they were not meant to eat…but you can greatly minimize the damage by following these steps. Hey, Baby! Can't touch this![141] ♪

- Put away anything tiny (marbles, dice, game pieces, thumb-tacks, paper clips, small jewelry, coins, hair pins).
- Make plastic bags inaccessible
  - o   If you use a plastic bag on the bathroom door knob for dirty diapers, get an over-the door towel hook and use that instead. Its too high for a baby or toddler to reach.
- Be wary of balloons
  - o   Burst balloons can pose a choking hazard.
- Plug electrical sockets securely with plastic safety plugs.
- Clip up any dangling curtain cords.
- Install baby gates at tops and bottoms of all stairs (be sure to install the ones that attach to the walls with hinges, not the pressure-mounted versions, as those can be pushed down).
- Tape down or tuck away electrical cords.
- Put a nonslip bath mat in tub.
- Put away (or completely dispose of) all chemical cleaners. Instead, use baking soda and vinegar—safe, effective, and edible.
- Install a safety lock on oven, medicine cabinet.
- Install safety lock on cupboards, drawers, garbage, toilet, etc.
  - o   This is optional, depending on the personality of your baby. For my oldest three, I didn't need these, but for—you guessed it—Maxwell, I needed them! I can't even count the number of times he played in the toilet. And, of course, Maxwell figured out how to open these as well. When Baby can open a cupboard even with the lock on it, use a strong rubber band to hold the two cupboard door-knobs together.[142] I used the kind that comes wrapped around broccoli, and that worked for keeping Maxwell

141 "U Can't Touch This" by M. C. Hammer, *Please Hammer, Don't Hurt 'Em,* 1990, Capitol (US) Records.
142 Carolyn Lauchlan, mom

out—whew! (He only ate from the garbage once, not bad, right? ☹)

- Never cook with the pot handles sticking over the side of the stove. Always turn them in so they can't be grabbed.
- Install a lock on your exterior doors that is up high (so toddler can't exit the premises unbeknownst to you).
- Keep second-story windows closed, especially if they have any objects in front of them that a toddler could use to climb on.
- Place fans out of reach.
- Put scissors up high, out of reach, in a hidden location, because a toddler will often seek out scissors to cut his hair or a sibling's hair. (We were always thankful it was just the hair.)
- Hide knives.
- Drape a folded towel over the top of all interior doors to prevent their being fully closed.[143] This stops tiny fingers from getting pinched and prevents toddlers from locking themselves in the bathroom. Yes, both scenarios have happened to us.
- Hide pens and permanent markers. Toddlers and young children can and will use them against you. They'll write on furniture, floors, and walls, their siblings...and themselves. Yesterday Terrek wrote "buger" (he meant booger) on Maxwell's leg. When I asked Max what those letters said, he replied, "it's my ABC's."

---

143 Ellen Ryan-Chan, teacher and mom

CHAPTER 31

Weaning the Baby

I'm so thirsty; I haven't had milk in a year.

P., AGE FOUR

Note: This weaning system is based on Mom going back to work at twelve months. If you need to return sooner, then refer to chapter 16, "Bottle- and Breastfeeding Together." If you are not returning to work, then there is no pressure to wean. Take your time and savor the joys of nursing for as long as you and your baby like.

Some babies wean themselves and lose interest in the breast. That was not the case with my babies. They all loved breastfeeding and so did I; in fact, it was a little sad to stop. I needed to initiate weaning, but it wasn't difficult because I did it very gradually, so it wasn't a shock to my baby or to my body.

First of all, I breastfed on demand right up to nine months old, then I cut out the night feedings. I continued to breastfeed during the day up until twelve months, the magical age when Mommy has to return to work (in Canada, anyway). By twelve months, the baby is eating a variety of foods and drinking water or breast milk from a sippy cup or a bottle. Now, it's easier to cut back nursing to mornings, bedtimes, and a few additional times during the day.

There is no need to stop breastfeeding before naps or to eliminate your daytime nursing entirely before you return to work. Continue nursing your baby. Some moms are extremely concerned about weaning their babies by their first day back to work. This is just not necessary. When you're away at your job, your absence naturally weans the baby. There is no need to struggle and deny him the breast beforehand; it will just cause unnecessary trauma. When you're at the office, your baby will notice you're not home and will drink more from the sippy cup or bottle when she is thirsty. Your body will automatically stop producing as much milk. It will all fall into place naturally, with no struggle required. You can continue to breastfeed in the mornings and evenings at home.

Be sure your nanny or day care provider does not put the baby down with a bottle for her nap. Even if you were breastfeeding at nap time before, here is a great chance to teach the baby to sleep without depending on the bottle. Since you're transitioning anyway, do both at the same time. Baby doesn't need to learn to fall asleep with the bottle and then have to be retrained to sleep without the bottle. Offer the bottle throughout the day and at meals and snacks. There will be plenty of opportunities for drinking milk; bedtime doesn't have to be one of them.

When I returned to work, I continued to breastfeed three times a day: first thing in the morning (try to do both sides before you leave for work or you may feel lopsided all day), immediately upon returning home from work, and right before bed. You may feel engorged the first day back at the job, but only for one day. Your body catches on quickly. I continued with nursing three times a day for about two months. Then I cut out the feeding right after work. We'd be busy having snacks and playing, so it was easy to distract my baby if he wanted to be nursed. The next feeding I cut was first thing in the morning. I'd get the baby up, and we'd be so busy getting ready for our day, it was again, easy to distract her from the regular nursing routine. The final feeding to go is the one right before bed. I ended that when my babies reached eighteen month by offering a delicious and nutritious smoothie right before bed (blend 1 cup of homogenized milk and one frozen banana). When she clamored to nurse before she went into her crib, I would simply say, "Oh, you don't need Mommy's milk. Your tummy is full with your delicious smoothie." My babies accepted this logical explanation and went to bed.

You can nurse your babies as long as you want. Breast milk is the best thing for them! I weaned my first three babies by the time they were eighteen months because I was pregnant again, and I felt that my body was getting drained. My lucky little fourth baby got breast milk much longer. I nursed him twice a day (morning and bedtime) until he was two and a half. It was such a special way to start and end each day together; we both treasured this special time.

Warning: once you stop nursing, your baby will forget about nursing completely within a couple of days! It will be like his mind was erased and all memories of nursing vanished. This seems sad when you have put in so much time, effort, and energy nursing for such a long time. It almost seems unfair! Rest assured that you did well. Your breast milk has nourished his little body and mind, and the good that you did while he was growing and developing will stay with him for the rest of his life. After you stop breastfeeding, your breasts will shrink down to smaller than your regular size. Get some nice new shapely bras. Your breasts have worked hard and are now ready for a rest! Bye-bye, big boobs.

CHAPTER 32

Day Care versus Nanny

> It's not my job to hold the bugs.
> —ME

Maternity leave goes by so unbelievably fast, and before you know it, the family needs to make child-care arrangements. While some mommies are ready for this and are excited to get back to their careers, this transition can be incredibly heart wrenching for others (like me!). It felt like the most unnatural thing to leave my baby. I dreaded going back to work (even though I love my job), and the thought of leaving my baby made me cry. I worried that my baby—who trusted me completely and for whom I was always there—would feel that I'd abandoned him. (I felt this way all over again with each subsequent child, although it did get easier each time, as I knew what to expect.) I can completely understand the rationale of moms who quit their jobs entirely when they have kids and decide to be a stay-at-home mom. The reality for most of us is that, for financial reasons, we have to go back to work. (Something about futures…pensions…university tuition? None of it seems to matter now—but one day it will.)

If you feel torn and sad about leaving your baby, take comfort in knowing that you both will adapt rather quickly and fall into the routine. You'll feel better about the change when you are comfortable with your child-care arrangements. Be sure to have these organized before you head back to work. Through the course of my four babies, I have somehow managed to try out a full spectrum of child-care arrangements, each prompted by specific reasons and needs we had at the time. In chronological order, we tried home day care, day care center, Montessori preschool, another day care center, and finally a nanny, and found advantages and disadvantages with each.

The main advantage of a day care center is the educational pro-graming often available there. The main plus of home day care is the cost (much cheaper). And the main advantage of a nanny is that the nanny makes life so much easier for Mom and Dad. At the end of my detailed accounts below is a chart to help you with the decision, and another outlining the contrasts between day care centers and private Montessori schools.

Let's face it—childcare is expensive! It hardly seems worth it to go back to work because you're shelling out half your salary for someone to watch Baby. Keep in mind that it's only for a few years. Before you know it, your child will be in school, so these child-care costs—while huge—are not forever. The number of children you have will dictate whether a nanny or day care is more affordable. Nanny care is approxi-mately the same as two children in full-time day care. So if you only have one child, day care is cheaper and home day care is even cheaper still. If you have three children, financially, a nanny is the better deal.

Home Day Care

With my first baby, Terrek, we moved into a new area soon before I had to return to work, so I had to scramble to find childcare. I was on waiting lists for stellar day care centers in our former city, but found the waiting lists were packed, and there were no open spaces for Terrek in our new city. So I researched home day care. This option can be terrific, but you must trust your child-care provider. She is on her own. One feature I like about day care centers is that the staff includes several teachers and child-care workers who are held accountable for their actions. They have a boss and coworkers always watching one another. Home day care—on the other hand—is headed by one per-son who is often a stay-at-home mom who has set up her own busi-ness. These moms are usually nurturing, kind, and dedicated, and if you find someone you trust and feel comfortable with, it could work out well. If you have a grandma available for snooping, you can verify! My mom stopped in to pick up Terrek early a few times and was able to observe a bit of what was going on. Usually, it was great. However, good old Grammy did catch a few factors not quite up to my standards—not dressing Terrek appropriately for the cold weather was one; giving him rides on top of a stroller canopy was another (yikes—unsafe). At least I was informed about these issues and could address them with the provider.

In home day care, the atmosphere is generally more relaxed than at a center, and the children get more free time to play. It's comfortable—your child is in a nice, cozy home instead of a school-like setting. Your child will be with a maximum of four other children and will get to know this small group well. Depending on the provider, the schedule will likely be more flexible as well—sometimes even for you. If you need to work late or are running late to pick up your kids, your home day care provider may be able to accommodate that, whereas day care centers usually cannot. (They close at a certain hour, and if you're late, you are charged steep fees.) Depending on your provider's policies, you may be able to send your child even if he is sick, although that means your child could make others ill, or vice versa, if other parents bring their sick kids, too. Accordingly, some home care providers have a no-sick-children rule.

Home care has other possible drawbacks, depending on the provider. It may not offer the kind of educational program a day care center can. The kids may mainly be watching TV, in a far less structured setting than a center's, though that may not be so bad: a comfortable, informal, safe place to play and relax may be just what your child needs. Do your research, find a provider you can trust, and home day care could be a great option for your family.

Day Care Center

When I had two children, I put my boys in a day care center. We actually tried out two. The first one was OK; the second one was a perfect fit! Be sure you visit your center and ask lots of questions before registering. The first center had a great program and facility, but was not especially receptive to my family's special food requirements (no red meat), and one of the teachers treated the kids with an abrupt and condescending manner that I didn't appreciate. The second center accommodated our food choices with respect and compassion, and the teachers were kind and considerate yet firm and consistent as well. It was such a good experience that even though I love our nanny, I send my kids to one year of preschool at the center part time.

The educational programs at day care centers are usually fantastic. Kids are mentally stimulated and busy all day. It's like kindergarten—they do crafts, sing songs, are taught cooperation skills, have outdoor play, learn letters and numbers, enjoy science activities, and more. Your child will make new friends and develop peer relationships. He will learn proper expectations and behavior for a kindergarten setting, such as sitting in a circle, lining up, and raising his hand. The children play outside and are well supervised. Staff are typically friendly and knowledgeable, well supervised, and professionally responsible, and they care about the kids. Day care centers both nurture and challenge children at the same time.

One drawback to day care homes and centers is the initial adjustment. (So sad and traumatic!) There will be a short phase in the beginning where your child screams and cries as if you have abandoned him in a terrible dungeon (and you cry in the car on your way to work), but it's short-lived. You'll have to leave your child in her hysteria and pretend that you are completely calm and relaxed for her sake, even though you are secretly panicking and contemplating quitting your job. Believe it or not, you and your child will both adapt quickly to this new separation. Soon, your child will be waving and saying, "Bye, Mommy! Love you. Have a good day!" The most amazing moment of the day will be when you pick your child up at the end. His little face will light up, and he'll come running, like you are long-lost loves, and he will shout, "Mommy!" and jump on you with a huge bear hug. I *love* this moment. ☺

One downfall with day care are the germs. Little kids put things in their mouths and aren't great at using a tissue when they have a runny nose. So little kids in day care get sick...a lot. (FYI: You can't send children to day care when they are sick, so you or your partner will have to take days off work, or you will have to call Grandma if she lives nearby.) While this is a huge pain, I'm told exposure to all these germs is building up your child's immune system, so maybe it's not so bad in the long run.

Another negative: the morning and afternoon rush of getting little ones out the door on time. Little ones need to be awakened, changed, and fed; to have teeth brushed and be dressed (in snowsuits in the winter), and then you have to stop and drop them off before you go to work. That's a hectic morning schedule, and it's so easy to be late and then be stressed. The afternoon pickup can also be hard to organize. By contrast, with a nanny, the mornings and evenings are less crunched.

As mentioned, too, day care center tuitions are quite expensive, a big burden for working families. But remember that childcare can be income-tax-deductible in Canada and the United States.[144]

Montessori Preschool

In my experience, a Montessori preschool is very similar to day care, with some specific differences. Both have an excellent educational program. The Montessori program is different in that it is very individualized, and the children work at their own pace on different tasks and skills. Both teach letters, numbers, science, and art. Both have music, story time, physical fitness, and outdoor time. And both offer comparable pricing. One vital curriculum difference: Montessori schools teach cursive writing before printing. The reasoning (as explained to me) is that cursive writing comes more naturally to a young child, a next step after scribbling, and is apparently easier. True or not, that practice seems of questionable benefit, as printing is what children learn in regular school, so printing is what they will need to be able to do when they get there. Additionally, as a teacher myself, I know that cursive writing, while beautiful, in our high-tech digital age is, sadly, becoming a thing of the past. Schools no longer teach it in most

---

144 http://taxes.about.com/od/deductionscredits/qt/child_care.htm

provinces in Canada or most parts of the United States.[145] Another note that may or may not matter to you: private Montessori schools do not use books about talking animals.

In many Montessori schools, lunch is not provided (some have catering; it varies from center to center), so you must pack one. That could be a plus for you if you prefer some control of your child's diet (day care menus' nutritional quality varies; factor it in when doing your research.) Yet packing your child's lunch is also one more job on your big daily mommy to-do-list. My Montessori school had refreshment time twice a day: morning and afternoon. Instead of snacks from home, the kids share a large selection of fresh fruits and vegetables. Each child brings a large portion of fruit or veggies once a week (for example, one cantaloupe or a bag of apples). The teachers cut the fruit, and the children share. I loved this plan, as it ensured that my kids were eating lots of fruits and vegetables throughout the day.

One great bonus to Montessori schools: they teach children to clean up after themselves! Kids learn to tidy up when finished with materials, right from the toddler age. It's an impressive responsibility lesson, and it works.

Pricing is pretty comparable between day care and Montessori, but Montessori days are shorter. So if you need extended childcare day, while this service is provided at Montessori schools, you will have to pay extra for this additional time. That can add up. You also don't get spring break and Christmas holidays included in your tuition, whereas with regular day care you do (minus legal national holidays). Montessori schools don't include summer in their regular program; if you are a teacher or planning a long summer vacation that may not matter (you save a lot of money and put them back in for the fall without worrying they'll lose their spots), or you can enroll your kids in the Montessori school's summer program (they call it a camp). In a day care center, you run the risk of losing your child's slot if you take him out for two months—something to consider.

145 http://www.washingtonpost.com/local/education/cursive-handwriting-disappearing-from-public-schools/2013/04/04/215862e0-7d23-11e2-a044-676856536b40_story.html

Montessori schools offer part-time programming, but require three consecutive days. Here is where I eventually ran into difficulty. Even though I loved the school and the teachers, I needed Tuesday/Thursday childcare for my toddler, Patrick, as Terrek was in part-time kindergarten and I wanted my boys home together on the same days. The Montessori school was not able to accommodate that. So my child-care journey continued, and I ended up loving my next day care center as well...maybe even more so!

Nanny

When I had three children, we hired our wonderful nanny. A nanny makes a busy life with kids significantly easier to manage. She is helpful around the house, able to help with cooking, laundry, and housecleaning, taking a load off the burdened schedule of working moms and dads. Having a nanny also eliminates the hectic morning drop-off and afternoon pickups. You can just leave the kids at home and the nanny walks them to school (or the bus stop). Another plus: when your child is sick and can't go to school or day care, the nanny is there; you don't have to take time off from work every time illness hits. A nanny can also be a wonderful alternate parent-figure offering kids another special relationship: she loves them, and they love her right back. Kids always need lots of love and attention, and when they get more love, it's a win-win.

Flexible scheduling is another clear benefit: if you and your partner have jobs where you have to work odd hours—weekends or evenings—a nanny is the way to go. She may also be available for babysitting if you and your husband need a date night!

Of course, to reap all these wonderful benefits, you need one crucial factor: the right nanny. You have to find one you feel utterly comfortable and happy with and whom you trust completely. It is especially important that your personalities mesh well if she is going to live with you. A live-in is usually more affordable than a live-out nanny, but a live-out may be more conducive to your lifestyle. Some families value their privacy and rhythms too much to have a stranger come live in their home. For us, live-in is a plus: my husband works a lot, so it's nice for me to have some adult company in the evenings with four crazy kids running around.

Our nanny is no trouble at all to live with—she actually reduces trouble, as she putters around and tidies up, even when not on duty. Creating this special relationship and getting the most out of your nanny experience is a two-way street. It's important that you are giving, welcoming, and kind to your children's caregiver. Treat her with respect and kindness, and she will do the same. If she works hard, include perks with the job—for example, pay for her dinners out, give her money for the dentist (very expensive, when not insured), and give her extra days off when you have some holidays from work.

Most people with nannies have a positive experience, though a few families do find their personalities just don't match, or they report such problems as a nanny being constantly on her phone or not being motivated. In my experience, these accounts are far more rare than the positive tales. Still, it's crucial to do your due diligence and interview carefully. A trial period is a good idea to make sure the nanny you hired is the one you want to keep.

TIPS FOR HIRING A NANNY

- Make a list of your expectations ahead of time. Put them in order of importance (e.g., caring individual, honest, reliable, knowledge of first aid, willing to do arts and crafts, able to swim, willing to do cooking and house cleaning, ability to speak native language).

- Make a list of nanny's duties (e.g., supervise children, walk children to school, change diapers, prepare formula, prepare meals, take children to park).

- Interview your potential nanny: first by phone, then, if possible, in person. (In-person interviews aren't feasible if you are sponsoring and hiring your nanny from overseas.). If you are able to meet in person, bring your children with you to see how they react to one another.*

Possible interview questions:
1. Describe your previous experience with children.
2. How would you handle a potential emergency?
3. What activities will you engage in with my child?
4. What is your discipline strategy?
5. Give an example of how you handled difficult child behavior in the past.
6. Why should I hire you over other nannies? What makes you stand apart?

- Ask for references.
* Source: Mary Anne Pangilinan

We completely got lucky with our nanny. I feel like we've adopted her as a member of our family. She is extraordinarily helpful and kind. I trust her to care for our children. And she maintains order in our household by being organized and efficient with laundry, cooking, and housework. She is astounding! She finds the time to do chores when the big kids are at school and the little ones are sleeping. The kids get to stay in the comfort of our home and to bond and interact with one another. I can get myself ready and go to work in the morning without a stressful drop-off, and, after work, I come right home, and the kids are already there. While I'm helping the kids with their homework and cuddling with the little ones, my wonderful nanny is starting dinner. Life is good with a good nanny!

One of my worries in hiring a nanny was socialization—that my kids wouldn't get the exposure to new friends and everyday interactions with peers that day care offered. To fill this gap, your nanny can bring your children to the park, where she will likely meet other nannies and can set up regular playdates, or in Canada, to a government-funded child play center (if you live close enough). Then again, when you have a big family, the kids can learn a lot interacting with one another! Neighbors and relatives with kids also provide plenty of opportunities.

Nannies also don't offer the rich educational exposure that day care can. Day care prepares your child for kindergarten. On the other hand, one may argue that kids spend their entire childhood in school, and a few extra years playing at home rather than in a classroom setting isn't going to hurt. "One" may have a point here!

Some mothers have expressed concern to me that their kids will love the nanny more than they love the mother. It makes sense when you think about it; the children spend more time with the nanny than with their own parents, so, of course, they will establish a special bond. I'll be honest. There have been moments when my little girl, Evelyn, will want our nanny instead of me. It does break my heart a little bit. However, usually she still wants me, and I understand that she's young and emotional. Most times, she's in the mood for Mommy, but sometimes she's in the mood for our nanny. She comes back around to me again. Keep in mind that the nanny is like a friend, buddy, and playmate as well as a caregiver. Sometimes kids want to be with their friends instead of their parents. However, a nanny is not a mother; it's not the same thing. There is no need to feel threatened or jealous. Just make sure you find some special time for one-on-one with your child, and you will maintain your special relationship.

When I think about the big picture, I reassure myself. If I consider my daughter's best interest, that partly entails getting love from more than just her dad and me. More love is good love. Additionally, keep in mind that a nanny is temporary. When she's older, our nanny will have moved on in her career to another job or her own family. But I will still be Evelyn's mom. Our nanny is a wonderful companion and friend for my little girl, but as my mother says, "No one can replace the mother." So don't stress, and do think about what's best for your kids. I don't know any kids who couldn't benefit from another person loving and caring for them.

Whichever child-care situation you decide upon, you will be surprised at how quickly you adjust to being a working mom after your maternity leave is over. You and your children will begin a new chapter in your lives. Nanny or day care can both be enriching choices. Do your homework and ponder what works best for your family. Use the following table to help guide your decision-making. Use a highlighter pen to mark the factors very important to you in yellow and the aspects you don't like with pink. You'll end up with a visual organizer to help pick the child-care option that best suits your needs.

DECISION-MAKING TABLE: CHILDCARE

HOME DAY CARE

ADVANTAGES	DISADVANTAGES
☑ Cheaper ☑ Relaxed, home environment ☑ Intimate, small group of peers ☑ Socialization opportunities ☑ Potentially more flexible hours/sick days	☒ Increased exposure to many kids who may be sick ☒ Difficult emotional adjustment for child (initially) ☒ One adult watching kids; you must trust person ☒ Hectic morning and afternoon pickups and drop-offs

DAY CARE CENTER

ADVANTAGES	DISADVANTAGES
☑ Educational Program ☑ Socialization with many peers ☑ Social behavior taught ☑ Preparing for kindergarten ☑ Several adults watching kids; staff always held accountable for actions	☒ Difficult emotional adjustment for child (initially) ☒ If your child is sick, you must make alternate arrangements ☒ Increased exposure to many kids who may be sick ☒ Inflexible schedule; set hours ☒ Hectic morning/afternoon pickups and drop-offs ☒ Expensive

NANNY*

ADVANTAGES	DISADVANTAGES
☑ Help for Mom and Dad— housework, cleaning, cooking	☒ Lack of socialization with peers
☑ Another "parent" to love children	☒ Lack of educational program
☑ Comfortable environment; child can stay at own home	☒ One adult watching kids; you must trust person
☑ Easier transition	☒ Expensive (if you have just one, equivalent if you have two, cheaper if you have three or more)
☑ Eliminate morning and afternoon hectic pickup/drop-off	
☑ Flexible schedule—can meet your needs (work late, sick child, etc.)	−/+ Nanny lives with you
☑ Consistent babysitter available if needed	Note: Nanny could be live-in (less expensive) or live-out (more expensive).
☑ Less exposure to germs and sickness	
☑ Flexible hours	
☑ Adjustment period to separation is less severe, as Baby is still in her own home	

DECISION-MAKING TABLE: DAYCARE CENTER VERSUS PRIVATE MONTESSORI SCHOOL

DAY CARE CENTER

ADVANTAGES	DISADVANTAGES
☑ Quality educational programming ☑ No extra charge for early morning/ late afternoon pickup ☑ No extra charge for Christmas holidays/ spring (March/Spring Break) ☑ Healthy meals included	☒ You may not remove your child to save money over summer holidays (you may take your child out, but will still be responsible for paying fees)

PRIVATE MONTESSORI SCHOOL

ADVANTAGES	DISADVANTAGES
☑ Quality educational programming ☑ May remove child for whole or part of summer (if you are a teacher, for example) so you can save money. Your child's spot is held for the fall. ☑ Healthy fruit and vegetable "refreshments" provided via a weekly parent donation system ☑ Train children to pick up after themselves at an early age	☒ Must pay for before- and afterschool care ☒ Must pay for Christmas holidays, spring break ☒ Don't use books with talking animals -/+May need to bring packed lunches (varies by location) -/+Still teach cursive writing

CHAPTER 33

Going from One to Two

Why are you crying?
—Me

Because Terrek is going to name me Ding-Dong.
—P., Age Four

Many people choose to have two children. It's a lovely number, and your baby has a sibling to grow up with, someone to play with, argue with, and love through thick and thin. It's a wonderful thing. It's also a manageable number of children: one child for each hand. The transition from one baby to two children is a bit challenging. I actually found it harder to go from one to two than from two to three or three to four. One to two is a big change. When you just have one baby, it's easy. All your attention is devoted to fulfilling one baby's needs. If your baby needs you, you are there. Your baby says, "Jump," and you say, "How high? How many times? One foot or two? Which direction? Whatever you want, Baby, because it's all about you!"

When you have a second baby, your new baby and your toddler will have very different needs, and often they will need you at the same time. Your toddler will have to learn to share you. You will find ways to juggle and give both what they need, but they will both have to learn to wait sometimes. That is good for them, although it may be hard for them to understand at first. The following are some tips to help ease your transition from one to two and to help juggle the demanding needs of an infant and a toddler.

You will need a few additional pieces of equipment, the first being a good double stroller. Get a double stroller that has an attachment to attach the infant car seat. This makes getting around so much easier. I also recommend the baby sling. If you didn't already get one with your first baby, it will come in handy now. It will allow you to hold and carry your baby around the house and still have an extra hand with which to tend to your toddler. Additional must-buy items are books that illustrate the story of a new baby coming to the family. This can help prepare your toddler for what is to come, and make him feel very special when the baby is here. There are so many wonderful books to choose from, such as *The New Baby* (Little Critter series) by Mercer Meyer[146] and *I'm a Big Sister* by Joanna Cole.[147] Just go to your local bookstore and have fun!

You will be more tired with your second baby than you were with your first because when you just had one baby, you could nap when your baby napped. Not so, anymore! You have a toddler to play with! You have double the children and that means double the needs to fulfill and double the energy you must exert. You still need rest—actually, more than ever. You will cherish your one nap a day (fingers crossed). The wonderful thing about babies is that they sleep. And a wonderful thing about toddlers is they still have a good, solid nap in the afternoon. The not-so-wonderful-thing about having an infant and a toddler is that it seems as though they conspire to rarely take their naps at the same time. If they happen to sleep at the same time—hallelujah—have a nap yourself, you tired mommy. But if they don't, at least try to catnap or rest a bit.

Napping gets more complicated when you have two. If you wake your baby early, put him down for a very early morning nap and then put your toddler down for a late afternoon nap. The late afternoon nap may coincide with your infant's afternoon nap. This would be ideal. However, unless you have an older sibling to walk to school, it

---

146 Mercer Mayer, *The New Baby* (New York: Random House, 1983).
147 Joanna Cole, *I'm a Big Sister* (New York: Harper Festival, 1997).

is very unlikely that you will be willing to wake up early to wake your infant up early. Sleep is too delicious for that!

Naptime is your goal. You will have to get creative with quiet activities during naptime. Use the following ideas to keep your toddler occupied and stationary while you grab a little shuteye as the infant snoozes. Note: you will never truly sleep so long as your toddler is awake. You'll always have to be on the alert to ensure your toddler isn't getting into mischief, but at least you can have a little quiet time and rest a bit, while your toddler is busy with a quiet and still activity.

1. TV—This is a time when the good old TV set comes in handy. I'd let my toddler crawl in bed with me, and I'd doze off while he watched Elmo and the baby slept. I'd wake up and groggily put on another episode until the baby woke up.
2. Library books—Fresh, new library books are always exciting. I'd get thirty of them and set up our at-home "library" and let my toddler sift through them while I took a snooze on the couch.
3. Tablets/iPads—We invested in a tablet for my kids—my toddlers loved to play with them, press buttons, etc. However, I found they work much better for older kids, as toddlers can get frustrated when they accidentally close their programs or when the program is stuck loading; you'll have to wake up to troubleshoot these types of problems. A little snooze on the couch while your child is playing with technology is possible, although it won't be a deep sleep.
4. Make a fort with couch cushions or a tent with a blanket and chairs. Put a blanket and pillow in there and let your toddler have some quiet time.
5. Art supplies—Set out crayons, Play-Doh, paper, and coloring books, and let your toddler go wild.
6. There are wonderful and educational websites where little kids can play on the computer. Again, it's usually better for older kids, but some are good for toddlers. Starfall.com and sesamestreet.org are two good ones.
7. LEGOs, blocks, and puzzles.

When you have an older child and an infant, things can get even more interesting. I trained my family to respect quiet time. Everyone in my house always understood that, after lunch, it was naptime for the baby, toddler (if they napped at the same time), and Mommy and quiet time for the older kids. During quiet time, they could do quiet activities in their room, like reading, coloring/drawing, and puzzles or playing with LEGOs. Tablets or iPads are extremely useful at this time, although I ensured they had reading time first. I always had the children close enough that I could hear them and would wake up if they got into mischief.

If you have help from parents or friends, this is where you should capitalize on your naptime. Have them take the older kids to the park so you can sleep when your infant sleeps. I depended on my naps during this early stage of motherhood. They were the difference between feeling completely tired, wrecked, and in a fog, and being able to function like a seminormal person.

When you have two kids, you will be especially happy that you sleep trained your baby, who is now a toddler. You will be so thankful that your toddler can now sleep through the night on his own. Waking with one baby throughout the night is difficult enough!

You're going to have to become an expert at doing things for your toddler while breastfeeding. I learned to breastfeed and make a snack, breastfeed and take the toddler to the potty, breastfeed and put on a Band-Aid, and breastfeed and put the toddler to bed. The most difficult task to achieve with one hand, while you are breastfeeding with the other, is putting a pair of pants on the toddler. While holding baby and breastfeeding with one hand, your other is trying to master the job of pulling up the toddler's pants. You are balancing on your toes, squatting at toddler's level, so you are already at a disadvantage because you're tippy. Kids this age are tippy simply because they are toddlers. They lose their balance, tip over, and grab you on the way down. You wobble, but hold on. He steps on the pant leg, so you can't pull the pants up, and it's hard to get the elastic waistband over his bottom. Then he steps on the other pant leg. Sometimes you end up pulling the pants on with both of the legs in one leg hole. Argh! It's frustrating! You'll see.

Expect some jealousy when you transition from one to two. I didn't notice it so much with two to three or three to four; the kids were used to sharing my attention by that time. But when I had my second baby, my firstborn, Terrek, a two-year old at the time, did show some jealousy. Of course he loved the baby, but he would also do mean things to the baby at times—pinching, pushing, and even biting. I scolded him and let him know this type of behavior was unacceptable. But I continued to give him extra love and praise, especially when he was gentle or sweet with the baby. I also made a big deal of telling Terrek just how much Patrick adored him and loved him. (At the time, this was news I invented, but it turned out to be 100 percent true!) Keep giving both of your kids love, and this phase will pass. Your older child will soon realize he now has a built-in playmate.

Your toddler also may go through an acting-like-baby phase. Terrek did when Patrick was born, and Evelyn dipped into this phase for a bit after Maxwell arrived. The toddler is fascinated and amazed by the new little life in the house. He also recognizes that this baby is getting a lot of attention for doing things that he has already mastered! The toddler is thinking, "Rolling on his tummy and holding his feet? That's a piece of cake! I can do that, too—I can do that really well. In fact, I can do that better than the baby! Watch me!" Don't worry about this phase. Your toddler will soon enjoy the fact that he is older and can do more things. Take this time to squeeze in your extra cuddles and give him the praise he is looking for. It reminds him he is still important and is still loved and special, and, besides, he will always be your baby anyway.

If you thought it was difficult to do simple things like take a shower and go to the bathroom when you just had one, know that it gets more difficult with two! When a new infant and a toddler are in the house, some toddlers do things to hurt the baby, intentionally or not. I couldn't leave Terrek and Patrick alone together for a second. The toddler would pinch the baby or play roughly with him. Once he picked his nose and put the booger in the baby's mouth. He even bit the baby on the hand a couple of times. If I had to go to the bathroom, one of them had to come with me. If I had to take a shower, the baby went in the bouncy chair in the bathroom and the toddler came in the shower with me. It takes some juggling, but once you develop a system, it becomes manageable. Some toddlers are very gentle with babies, and you won't have any problems, but if you do, don't worry; it is normal, and it will pass.

Perhaps the largest challenge is when both baby and toddler cry at the same time in the night. To whom do you go first? It's time to wake up your darling husband. You go to one, while Daddy goes to the other. Of course, they'll both want you. That is the way it goes. At least it's nice to be needed. You are the chosen one! You'll do juggling and go back and forth. Persevere! You'll get there.

Going out and about with a baby and a toddler can take a bit of getting used to. You'll have to learn to juggle. Although, there's no need to enroll in clown school. Here are a few ways to help manage a baby and a toddler out in the world (believe me, it will feel good to get out!).

- Wear the baby sling. You can use it to help carry your toddler as you carry the baby car seat with the other hand, if you are going somewhere that you can't take the stroller. You can use it to help hold the baby while you hold your toddler's hand. (You may equate yourself to a packhorse or a donkey in these situations; it won't be the last time!)
- When getting the baby out of the vehicle and reaching in to undo the buckles, teach your toddler to hold your leg once he's out of the vehicle.[148] That way you can feel him and know he isn't wandering around in the parking lot.
- Enroll in free activities for your toddler to entertain him so you can sit back and hold the baby (for example, at the library or in playgroups).
- Consider a backpack diaper bag (size large—you'll need it to hold stuff for the baby and toddler). It keeps your arms free to hold and manage your kids.

Now you're not just a mom of one, you're a super-busy mom of two. You have given your children the best possible gift: a sibling. They will learn to enjoy each other; they will develop their own relationships. This is only the beginning!

---

148 Shalimar Santos-Comia, RN and mom

CHAPTER 34

Potty Training

This potty seat is broke. Nothing came out.
—T., AGE TWO

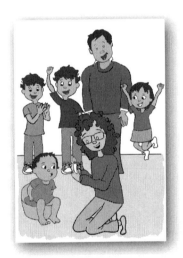

I have gotten potty training down to a science. If you stick to my program, training should take about one week, for both days and nights. No "big kid" diapers required. It works. But as with sleep training, you must have conviction and stick to it. In about a week, you and your child will be entering a new phase. It's so exciting and liberating! No more diaper changes!

The optimal age for potty training, in my experience, is two for girls and two-and-a-half for boys. You can watch for signs of readiness;

your child may be ready earlier or later. Such signs include being interested in the toilet, noticing when she pees or poos, asking to have
her diaper changed, wanting to sit on the toilet, and talking about the
toilet. My oldest son did not show any signs of readiness, but I just
decided to potty-train him anyway at two-and-a-half, and it worked.

Be wary of potty-training methods outlined by diaper companies.
Remember, their objective is to sell more diapers. If you potty-train your
child quickly, you won't be buying any more diapers. My method for
training is cold turkey. Get rid of diapers and "training pants" forever!
No turning back. If you waver and go back to diapers or "training pants"
for naps and outings, you will confuse your child, and potty training will
take longer. You won't need those, but you will need these items:

- Potty seats for all your toilets
- Potty (portable)
- Step stools for each bathroom
- Folding potty seat (to keep in the diaper bag for outings—optional)
- Lots of big-boy or big-girl underwear
- Candle and matches
- A mop
- Plastic tablecloths or sheets (two)
- Cloth training pants (for sleeping)
- Patience (plenty)

Plan to start potty training when you and your kids can be home
together for a week (optimally) or a long weekend (like Easter) without
having to go anywhere. It's also helpful if the weather is warm, so you
won't have to dress your child in layers. If you can whip off the undies
quickly to make it to the toilet on time, you'll have more success. Get
rid of your diapers. Tell your child that he is big now and doesn't need
diapers anymore. Be very excited about this. Your child will catch on to
your enthusiasm. Dress your child in the big-kid underwear. Children
are excited about wearing these. They can even be involved in buying
these beforehand and picking out ones they like. Start with confining
your child to areas of the house that do not have carpet. Keep your

child off the couch. (During potty training, Maxwell told our house guests, "Max not allowed on couch.") Your child will have accidents at the beginning, so be ready. Play on the bare floor that's easy to clean, and outside in the backyard.

Keep the portable potty in the same room as you are in so you can get to it fast. Your child will learn to go to the big toilet soon, but for the initial training, I recommend keeping the potty nearby. Your child will learn to "hold it in" quickly, but at the beginning, it's hard to do. Kids need to find and develop the squeezing muscles. After a few days, take away the potty and have your child use the regular toilet.

Some people say you shouldn't have a potty in the same room because the child will get used to it and instead should learn to use the regular toilet right from the start. I disagree; in my view, the in-room portable is a crucial piece of the training program. Your toddler will have more success with an immediately accessible potty. Again, this in-room setup is not permanent; it is only for two to three days, so your child will not have time to start relying on it. After you take it away, your child will already have got the feel for holding pee in a little and will be more successful at holding it during their mad dash to the real toilet. (You can also take the potty outside to the backyard with you, put it in the wagon when you go to the park…you get the idea!)

At first, your child won't tell you when she has to pee because she won't know. It's a surprise to her when she spontaneously starts peeing. It's your job to sit her on the toilet at regular intervals—every twenty minutes to half an hour. Sit her there and suggest she try pee-ing. Sometimes it takes quite a while for the pee or poo to come. Entertain your child by telling stories, looking at books, saying nursery rhymes, counting, or playing patty-cake. Of my four toddlers, it was Maxwell who really took his sweet time to pee and poo. Distracting him so he would sit on the toilet long enough to succeed was impor-tant. For his favorite diversion, whoever took Maxwell to the toilet would act out made-up stories about him and his siblings using their fingers as characters, as in a puppet play.[149] You can also try turning on the tap slightly and hope the trickling sound gets the pee-stream

---

149 Rose Reyes, nanny

moving. After your child is finished sitting on the potty, praise him for trying, and if he actually goes in the potty, have a party! Jump around and cheer, and shout for joy. This is a big deal in his little world. Make it fun and make him feel positive and proud. Instead of using a sticker rewards chart, I always sang "Happy Potty" to my toddlers and let them blow out a candle.[150] (Sing "Happy Birthday" but change the words.) They absolutely love this. It makes the achievement special and provides incentive so he'll want to use the potty again.

If your child has an accident, don't scold her. Just let her sit in the wetness and feel uncomfortable for a few minutes. Take your time to clean up the mess, then clean her up and change her. Remain positive.[151] Say things like, "Oh dear, you had an accident. That's too bad. Next time, go to the potty as fast as you can, and pee in the potty, OK?" If you see your child starting to pee in her pants, clap loudly and shout to distract her, in hopes of stopping her midstream, and scoop her up and sit her on the potty. If she gets any in the potty, it counts as a success. (This works for puppies, too, by the way.)

After a couple of days, you won't need the potty with you in each room anymore. Your child will now be able to make it to the big toilets in the actual bathrooms. It's handy to have your step stool and potty seat set up and in the ready position for when your toddler has to go. Soon, your child will be telling you when he has to pee and poo, and you can stop the regular proactive "seating"; you can gradually phase this out.

After a few days, you will need to start getting out and about in the world. Do not revert to diapers in the car out of fear of ruining your child's expensive car seat. Instead, put a towel-lined plastic bag on the car seat just in case. I did that but only needed it once (Maxwell). What I did need in the car was to keep the potty seat in it.[152] It's a necessity, and you will be very thankful for it. Your toddler is just learning to hold it when she has to pee. She will not be able to hold it for very long, so when you're driving along and she shouts, "I go pee! I go pee!" you can just pull over and use the potty in the privacy of your own car. No need

---

150 Shalimar Santos-Comia, RN and mom
151 http://www.babycentre.co.uk/a4399/abc-of-potty-training
152 Mary Anne Pangilinan, mom

to find a parking spot and a public washroom facility, cart your toddler and other kids with you, and cause an enormous delay to your travels. That all may just end up with your toddler peeing her pants en route. It's faster and smarter to have a potty seat on call at all times in your car. Keep some tissue and hand sanitizer on hand as well, along with some water to rinse out the potty seat to prevent unpleasant smells on your road trip. You'll be able to share funny anecdotes with your spouse about who had to dump the little turd behind a tree! ☺

You can't train a toddler to sleep through the night without peeing, can you? Yes, you can! Do it at the same time as potty training during the day. Parents always underestimate their toddlers; you'll be surprised to know it is easy to potty-train your child, even at night and nap time. Do not use the training or "big-kid" diapers; these will send mixed messages, your toddler may come to rely on them, and potty training will take a lot longer.

Instead, for the first little while *only* (a few days to one week), use cloth training pants. You can find these wherever you buy cloth diapers (e.g., Sears). Cloth training pants feel like underwear, so your child will sense consistency when potty training. When they're wet, they feel uncomfortable, unlike disposable training pants, which are very absorbent and feel dry even when they're wet. I used the cloth ones to save on laundry time (washing sheets is a pain), but I didn't use them for very long. I didn't need to. Toddlers hate the feeling of peeing in these and quickly learn to wake up to pee in the toilet at night or learn to wait until morning to "go."

Cloth training pants are not 100 percent effective. In fact, they can be quite leaky. They help keep the bed dry some of the time; other times not. I think it depends on the angle at which the peeing occurred in relation to the position of the pants. For the accidents, be prepared. When I make my toddler's bed, I put a plastic tablecloth or plastic sheet over the mattress and under the sheets.

Also double-make the bed.[153] Make the bed as you usually would: put a plastic sheet over the mattress, then bottom sheet, top sheet and blanket. Then put a second plastic sheet over the blanket, then

---

153 Ellen Ryan-Chan, teacher and mom

another bottom sheet, then a top sheet and a blanket over that. Now you have two sets of bed linens on the bed, separated by a plastic sheet. When one is soiled in the night, just rip if off from the second plastic sheet up, revealing a nice, clean second set of sheets and blankets underneath. Bingo: no fumbling around to remake the bed in the middle of the night.

To train your toddler to stay dry in bed, follow these steps: First, take your toddler to pee right before bed and keep it positive. (Forcing never works and just makes her resist.) Build it into your routine. Toddler must pee or at least have "a good try" before bed; then she gets to read a special book with you. If your toddler refuses to pee before bed, remind her of her expectation: "pee first, then book." If your child still refuses; do not read her a book, put her right to bed without the book. Your child will likely get upset by this, but it's important not to give in. Next time she will understand her job is to pee first, then she gets to have book time with you. Alternately, you could try an "everybody pees" approach. This is great if your toddler has older siblings, but parents can participate as well. Everyone line up and pee one by one, including your toddler[154]. She will feel included and grown up.

After she uses the toilet, right before bed, explain to your child, "We don't pee in the bed; we pee in the toilet. If you have to go pee in the night, wake up your body and call Mommy. I'll take you to pee in the toilet." Put on the special "nighttime underwear" (cloth training pants), and go to bed.

Then, before you go to bed, around ten o'clock or so, take your toddler for a "dream pee." To complete a "dream pee" successfully, scoop your sleeping toddler up from his bed, trying not to wake him. Sit him on the toilet, still cuddling him so he stays asleep, and whisper in his ear, "You're on the toilet now. Go pee." He will pee (usually), and then you carry him back to bed. For some kids, the dream pee is the key to keeping dry the rest of the night and for toilet-training success (true for my oldest two sons).

This tactic doesn't work with some kids (my daughter) and for some children, it only sometimes works (my youngest son). Note: it

---

154. Marian Orleans, mom

may take a while for the dream pee to click (Maxwell). When I first attempted the dream pee with him, Maxwell would just sit there, not pee, and look at me with a confused expression, wondering what we were supposed to be doing. After some time with successful potty training, Maxwell began to associate the toilet with peeing, and then the dream pee became effective on some days. It was hit and miss for him. I learned to attempt the dream pee with Maxwell, only if he did not pee before going to bed.

When I attempted to take Evelyn to the toilet at night, during potty training, Evelyn would get so mad! For dream-pee-resisters, you're better off skipping it. Evelyn would wake if she had to pee, or she would just hold it all night and pee on the toilet first thing in the morning. When I attempted the dream pee with Evelyn, she would have nothing to do with the measly problem of peeing interfering with her beauty sleep. She refused to cooperate. As soon as I'd sit her on the toilet, she'd say, "No pee! No want to! I go back bed!"

If your toddler cries in his sleep, it may seem like he is having a scary bad dream, but it's probably your signal that he has to pee! Go to him, pick him up, and sit him on the toilet. He will most likely pee. You can gently whisper to him, "Pee out the bad dream,"[155] and he will. When he's finished, put him right back to bed, and he'll go right back to sleep. In fact, I've found that bad dreams and night-crying are almost always remedied with a night trip to the toilet, a trip your child can wake himself in order to make, independently, around age six or seven.

In the morning, take your toddler to the toilet right away. When she has a dry night, cheer, dance, and have a happy little celebration. If your toddler wakes up wet, do not scold her. Instead, say, as you did when she missed the portable toilet, "Oh dear, you had an accident in your bed. That's too bad." Take your time and calmly change the sheets and clean up your child. Say, "Next time, if you have to pee in the night, wake up your body and call Mommy. I will take you to pee in the toilet." These steps work. In approximately one week your toddler will be toilet-trained in the day *and* at night (with the occasional accident). Really.

---

155 Susan Waite, mom

This system worked for my children and for other moms I know who used a cold turkey approach (stopping diapers altogether—even at night). For moms afraid to take that risk, potty training took a lot longer and was frustrating.

Some children wet the bed well into their childhood years. I don't know what potty-training method their parents used, so I can't comment. Sometimes an underlying medical condition or other bodily or developmental factors are the reason. My advice is to try my potty-training system, and give it a week or two, or three at the most. (Maxwell took two weeks). If it is not working, your child might require special attention or maybe just more time. See your pediatrician for specific advice if you are concerned. Don't panic. Everything happens in time, and your child may just not be ready yet.

FYI: the best way to wipe a toddler's bottom is to have him put his hands on the floor after getting off the toilet. This automatically sticks his rear in the air and you have a clear view and access to wipe him clean easily (think the downward-dog yoga pose). He looks completely ridiculous, but never mind! Additionally, always let your toddler flush the toilet. This is tremendous fun for him! (If you accidentally flush for him, he'll get mad…just wait and see!)

Additional Tip 1: When potty training your toddler, don't ask him: "Do you need to go pee?" The answer will always be "no," and then an accident may follow. Instead say, "It's time to go pee," and take your toddler to the toilet.

Additional Tip 2: Avoid giving your toddler big drinks of water before bed. If they are really thirsty, try just a little sip or two.

If Your Child Regresses

After my first three were potty trained, we never looked back. It was "full toilet ahead!" However, with little Maxwell, we did have some unfortunate setbacks. He was fully trained; according to plan, and then, two months later, he started having frequent accidents. Maybe because he was too busy and distracted to think about it, until it was too late. I had already phased out the candle and song, so maybe he lost interest. Maybe it was because I wasn't as diligent checking in with him, as I had been with the others. Whatever the reason, if this happens to your child, don't focus negatively on the incidents. Don't scold, don't pretend to cry, don't wallow in despair. (All of these actions will just perpetuate the negative occurrences of peeing/pooing in pants). What you need to do is revisit the potty training regime. Check in with him often; bring him to the potty regularly even if he says he doesn't have to go. For bedtime: insist upon the dream pee and consider bringing back the cloth training pants. When he has success in the toilet, cheer and bring out the old candle and "Happy Potty" song again. Make it positive, and a big deal. He'll enjoy this attention, and you'll be back on track.

CHAPTER 35

Transition to the Big-Kid Bed

Can I go on a garbage truck when I'm an astronaut?
—T., AGE FOUR

The big-kid bed is a big move for a toddler; most will embrace this new change with gusto (like my sons did), and others will cling to their old ways like a baby monkey (like my daughter did). Either way, it's a transition from baby to child, so it is special. The ideal age for transitioning out of the crib is approximately two years old. This is when my sons had learned to climb out of the crib, so they needed to get into a bed as soon as possible, before they fell on their heads. My daughter loved her crib and did not want to sleep in the big-girl bed in her new room. I wouldn't have minded delaying, but I was pregnant and due in a few short months, so I knew it was time. The baby would soon need the crib. If you are expecting, it's especially important to transition your toddler out of the crib at least two months before the baby comes so your toddler won't resent the baby for having "stolen" his bed. Two months is long enough for your toddler to forget all about the crib before its new occupant arrives.

With my boys, it was easy. I just took away the crib and showed them their new big-boy beds. I put safety rails on the sides of the beds so they wouldn't fall out. Since they were strong-willed and resisted going to bed at times, I also put a baby gate on the door of their room to prevent nocturnal rambles. That worked well, although I did find each of them asleep at the door on the floor a few times. You also must babyproof your toddler's room so they don't get into mischief when out of bed. (Once I came in to find petroleum jelly smeared all over Terrek—in his hair, on his clothes and face, all over the walls and shelves. FYI, petroleum jelly is very hard to clean off! Don't leave it within a toddler's reach. Terrek went on our holiday with a crazy, greasy hair-do.)

After about six months, the baby gate was no longer useful, as Terrek learned to climb over it, and Patrick and Maxwell both busted it down like a bulldozer (Patrick actually broke it). My daughter, Evelyn, did not need a baby gate on her door at all. When it was time to go to sleep, she simply stayed in her bed and went to sleep…imagine that! What a thought.

Evelyn did not embrace the whole big-kid bed idea. She cried and longed for the familiar comfort of her crib. It broke my heart to evict her for the new baby who would need it. So I found a solution that could satisfy everyone. I borrowed an extra playpen from my sister and set it up in my daughter's room. It worked like a charm. She appreciated the security of having four small walls around her while she slept. She eventually learned to climb in and out of it on her own, but that was no problem because she could do it safely, and when it was time to sleep, she stayed in it.

During this transition time, it's fun to get special new blankets and a pillow for your toddler—time to ditch the much-loved sleep sack. Make her new big-kid bed her own, a place to be proud of. If your toddler tosses off her blankets in the night, then I suggest dressing her in "snugglies" for bed: cozy clothes that are a bit too big so she can wear them over her pajamas (e.g., a fleece top and jogging pants). That way, she won't wake you in the middle of the night because she's cold and can't find her blanket. She will sleep soundly, warm, cozy, and snuggly in her snugglies!

CHAPTER 36

Temper Tantrums

> Don't want it. Don't like it. No wear
> it. I want my Spider-Man suit.
> —P., Age Two

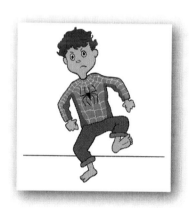

The terrible twos live up to their name. They're the most difficult age I've encountered so far as a parent. Before I had kids, when I witnessed screaming toddlers who were having a hairy fit in a public place, I must admit I judged the parents. I looked at them and thought, "What terrible parents. I'd never let my child behave like that. It's despicable." Oh, my naïve days…I knew nothing of the terrible twos at that time. And my, oh my, now I know all too well how it feels to be the parent in that situation! I've had to carry my kids (one in particular) kicking and screaming for the whole world to see at various public places (movie theater, grocery store, mall, parking lot, day care) and, of course, at home. I have dealt with ridiculous hairy fits based on something that makes no sense at all to a reasonable human being. To toddlers, it's an emotional, life-changing problem for which they just can't see a plausible solution, and their little world is crashing down around their heads. They cry, scream, go limp, go stiff, hold on to furniture for dear life, hide under a chair, hit, kick, and stomp. (If you're lucky, they don't do all of these at the same time.) It's extremely embarrassing.

The temper tantrum age usually hits in the twos, continues into the threes, and tapers off by the fours. If parents handle them correctly, tantrums should no longer happen by kindergarten.[156] Some kids hit the tantrum phase earlier, some later, and some not all (lucky parents). My mother swears that neither my sister nor I had tantrums. These temper fits vary in degrees of severity. Tantrums are just *in* some kids; it's how they react to their world.

Evelyn, as a terrible two, had some tantrums, but hers were mild compared to my sons'. Oh, my goodness—crazy, wicked fits, especially my second son, Patrick! His blowups were intense, and he didn't care where he was or who was around when he erupted. I found some solace when I heard that toddler tantrums prove a child has a real mind of his own (evident!). If taught properly, these strong-willed toddlers may grow into the kind of teenagers who don't follow the crowd.[157]

However, children who throw fits without intervention may not learn to behave respectfully or make good choices on their own. Ronald G. Morrish, educator and behavior consultant, emphasizes that parents need to guide these stubborn kids on how to behave appropriately. He explains stubbornness can evolve into a positive trait when parents learn not to give in to tantrums but instead help direct their child's behavior.[158]

Getting through this phase is trying and very difficult. With most tantrums, there's nothing you can do to stop them from happening,

---

156 Ronald G. Morrish, parenting expert, educator and behavior consultant

157 Ronald G. Morrish, in a parenting lecture in November 2011. Morrish is the author of *Secrets of Discipline* (Fonthill, Ontario: Woodstream Publishing, 1997).

158 Ronald G. Morrish, parenting expert, educator and behavior consultant

and you have to ride them out. But, as with my potty- and sleep train-ing plans, consistency is the key for effectively dealing with them. Never, not even once, can you give in to a tantrum. If parents do that, even 10 percent of the time, Morrish says, kids are learning to con-tinue with this behavior.[159]

I've tried many different strategies with my kids, and I've come to the realization that you cannot reason with a toddler in the middle of a tantrum. It's not possible; he is not in the right mind-set. You'll have to let the tantrum pass and speak to him calmly later about how he should have behaved differently.

While the child is having a fit, do not be sucked into his emotions. You have to remember that your child is not your peer. You are the adult. It is tempting to engage in an argument with your toddler or get angry and start yelling at him. Neither approach is effective or helpful. You need to disengage yourself from the turmoil and realize your child does not have control of his emotions. You, however, are the adult, and you know it's possible to maintain control of your emo-tions. Think of your toddler as a person who is not in his right mind, a person who does not know what he is doing. You need to take a step back. Remember to be patient. Sometimes I would whisper to myself, "Patience, patience, patience." This helped me to remember that I was dealing with a small child. Of course, there are times when it is necessary to raise your voice, but there is a difference between raising your voice in a firm, controlled manner and yelling, screaming, and popping a blood vessel. You have to remain in control because your child is out of control when he is having a tantrum. You must shake it off![160] ♪

In the heat of a tantrum, you also need to be firm and consistent. I said things like, "This is not how we behave. I will speak to you when you calm down." I would remove my child from the situation and put him in a time-out, so he could calm down in a quiet, neutral spot. All my children would sit in the time-out spot except Patrick. Sometimes they would cry, yell, or shout, "I'm done! I'm done!" repeatedly. I

159 Ronald G. Morrish, parenting expert, educator and behavior consultant
160 "Shake It Off," Taylor Swift, *1989*, 2014, Big Machine.

wouldn't talk to them until they were quiet, and they understood this. When they were quiet, I knew they were ready.

Patrick would not sit in time-out. I would put him there, and he would get up and follow me around the house. He would try to attach himself to me somehow by clinging to my leg, or climbing on my back. He made it very difficult to ignore him. So I had to resort to bringing him up to his room and closing the door. I made sure he was safe, and I was close by (wanting to cry myself). He would stay at the other side of the door, kick it, and continue screaming. I sat on the opposite side of the door and quietly held it closed. I found (after trying many different strategies) that this situation is what he needed to calm down. He needed to know I was serious, that he had to stop crying and screaming if he wanted me to talk to him and pay attention. He needed to stay in one place and settle. And I did not want to give him attention for his negative behavior. (I tried the sometimes-recommended tactic of holding and hugging him until he calmed down, but that backfired: He thrived on my attention and would push and kick and get worse and worse. His tantrums were shorter when I removed myself from his presence.)

It was always very difficult for Patrick to get out of a tantrum mind-set, and waiting took a great deal of patience on my part. He could carry on for forty minutes, sometimes in full-fledged fit mode. As difficult as it was, we got through it. As he grew older and more mature, his tantrums became less frequent and less severe. He learned what to expect when he was having a tantrum. When he was four, he would sometimes have the odd tantrum for old time's sake. He would then sit in time-out. (Hallelujah! He finally got it.) Now, I'm so proud of my six-year-old son who is level-headed and mature for his age. Patrick, the same tantrum-prone child, received the Integrity Award in his kindergarten class, last year, for always making good choices and doing the right thing. I can now see that my firm, consistent approach worked and is working.

After a tantrum, when my child was calm and sad, I would go to him, and we'd have a talk. He would have to say sorry to me. I always wanted him to understand that this behavior was unacceptable, and he must apologize for acting like that. (If he wasn't ready to apologize, then we weren't ready to talk.) He had to explain what he was sorry for. We'd talk about what just happened, and I would ask him why he was sorry. My child learned to identify something that went wrong. Then we would talk about how he could have behaved differently. What should he have done? I would also listen to him.

I also taught my child to identify his emotions. And it was important to me that he felt heard. I would say something like, "I understand you were mad because you didn't want to leave the movie theater, but it was time to go home." I would keep it simple, firm, and neutral. I made sure he knew I still loved him, no matter what. My oldest son learned to remove himself and give himself his own time-outs when he was feeling upset. I think he got to this awareness because of all the talking about feelings that we did as he was growing up. He learned to recognize that he was feeling angry or frustrated, and he knew that he would calm down with a little quiet time, all by himself. He would read books or draw and just rest and have peace for a while. He would come back, like his old self again, refreshed and happy.

There is no quick fix for temper tantrums; many children go through this phase. Some strategies work sometimes, depending on the personality of the child and the circumstances surrounding the fit. Out of the many tactics I've tried, the most effective include removing the power, distracting, picking your battles, extra love, and being proactive with my child's needs. Always remember to give lots of extra positive attention when your child is behaving well.

Removing the power[161] involves taking the power struggle off the table and allowing the power to fall to the toddler. The toddler feels like she is in control of the decision-making and the problem solving, while the parent actually maintains the control. For example, my sister was preparing a bubble bath for her daughter, and her daughter had a tantrum about the bubbles. She didn't want any bubbles in the tub. My sister removed the power by saying, "OK, how should we get the bubbles out?" This diffused the tantrum by switching gears for the child, who then had the power and had to figure out how to scoop

---

161 Ellen Ryan-Chan, teacher and mom

the bubbles out of the tub and into the sink with a bucket.[162] She proceeded to have an agreeable bath. Note that the parent did not give in to the child's wrath, but she successfully diverted the tantrum.

Distracting and redirecting works especially well when your toddler is young. If he is freaking out about a toy that broke and nearing an emotional breakdown, you could divert him by shouting, "Oh look, I see the garbage truck!" Or, "Look at the bird outside. I think it's trying to find a worm." Young toddlers will be fascinated with the new discovery, drop the broken toy, and forget about it. Be sure to hide it when they're not looking! This is a very positive way to switch gears and start fresh.

Picking your battles can avert certain tantrums. When you know your child well, you can predict what types of things may set him off. You must stick to some of the choices you make for your kids (eating healthy, bedtime, safety rules, manners, time to go, etc.). But for other, less serious, choices you could just forfeit the win and let your child have his way *before* a tantrum occurs (never after or during). For example, Patrick went through a serious superhero costume phase where he wanted to wear his Spider-Man suit everywhere. If I suggested he wear normal clothes, I could see him getting tense and emotional; I could feel the storm brewing! So I thought to myself, "What's the big deal if he wears a Spider-Man suit for our professional family photo? He actually looks pretty cute, and we'll laugh about this in years to come." (We do.) So I let him wear it. He wasn't hurting anyone, and he was happy as pie. Tantrum avoided.

Extra love is just what children need sometimes. A child could be acting up because he feels left out. Be sure you are paying enough attention to your child on a day-to-day basis. Take time out of the hectic business that is the life of a working parent and play with your child. Read to her, make popcorn together, and snuggle on the couch. Tell her often how much you love her. Tell her what a good kid she is and how proud you are of her. Let her "overhear" you telling others how good she is. This will make her feel good, and if anything, she'll want to live up to that and will work harder to be better. Do not give

---

162 Ibid.

your child more love in the middle of the tantrum. She may take this as permission to continue the tantrum. Give your child more love when she is behaving well.

Being proactive with your child's needs is essential to avoiding many preventable tantrums. My children were always worse if they were overtired or hungry. It was important for us to stick to a regular bedtime and nap schedule. I knew that if my toddler missed her nap or was very late for her nap, I was in for a cranky-pants kid! If we were up too late the night before, the next day, we paid for it with crying over silly things and getting disproportionately upset. Kids can't effectively handle their emotions when they are very tired. They need regular sleep to be on their best behavior. That also goes for hunger. A hungry child is a grumpy child. Pack snacks, and eat at regular mealtimes, and your child will be happier.

Temper tantrums are enormously difficult to handle for a parent. Remember that this behavior is a phase, and it will pass. Try what works for you and your child, but do be consistent. Above all, keep control of your own emotions, and your child will learn to respect you and will eventually model you. Good luck!

CHAPTER 37

Schedules and Routines

I'm the motor, but still, don't sit on my head, OK?
—P., Age Four

Your baby's needs change as she grows, so her schedule and routine will change as well. At first, there is no schedule; there shouldn't be. Your baby will dictate when she eats, sleeps, and poops. As your baby grows, she will build her timetable and routine. Pay attention to her cues and let it happen naturally. When your baby is older—and definitely when she is a toddler and a young child—a schedule is very important. With a schedule in place, your child will get enough sleep, be able to function properly throughout the day, and be more manageable because she will know what to expect. She will be trained. That's especially necessary when you have more than one child. When you have them all on a schedule, maintaining and keeping everyone happy is much easier.

Sleeping is very family-specific. Some families sleep in later in the morning, and some wake early. Some families stay up later, and some go to bed early. Often it depends on work and school hours. Your family sleep patterns will influence your baby's sleep schedule, naturally. Keep in mind that babies and children need a lot of sleep in order to grow, be healthy and behave properly. Here are guidelines for typical natural sleep patterns.[163]

---

163 http://www.webmd.com/parenting/guide/sleep-children

RECOMMENDED AMOUNT OF SLEEP FOR YOUR BABY*	
BABY'S AGE	HOURS OF SLEEP NEEDED PER DAY
1-4 weeks old	15-16
1-12 months old	14-15
1-3 years old	12-14
3-6 years old	10-12
7-12 years old	10-11

* http://www.webmd.com/parenting/guide/sleep-children

We are an early rising family: Mom and Dad get up for work, and the kids go off to school. The children wake up around six-thirty in the morning and are in bed by eight o'clock in the evening. Keep this in mind when you read the following information. The times may be different in your household, but the number and approximate timing of the naps will likely be similar.

Newborn: As a newborn, your child will make up her own schedule. Actually, at first there is no schedule. Your baby will sleep a lot, around the clock, and will also want to nurse a lot, around the clock. You can't hold newborns to an exact routine. They have specific needs; they have tiny bodies, and they are just figuring out what it feels like to be hungry or cold or to have to burp. In your tummy, your baby's needs were constantly met at all times. So have patience; a schedule will come, but not yet.

Two Months: There is still no real schedule. However, your baby will sleep more during the night now and be awake more during the day. My first two, Terrek and Patrick, continued night feedings every two hours until about nine months. Terrek continued waking up frequently in the night because he was wet. (Thus I changed him, and nursed him back to sleep). I used cloth diapers during the night with him—oops—see more about that in chapter 19, "Diapering Baby." And Patrick just *loved* eating (he was adorably chubby). Evelyn and Maxwell would wake up only one to two times a night after two months.

Three Months: Life with your baby will start getting easier around the three-month mark. She will start to sleep for long stretches at night, maybe even the entire night. (This won't last, so don't get used to it!) She will not be as fussy and will be more aware of her surroundings. Your baby is still not on a set daily timetable. She eats on demand and sleeps a lot. She will feed a lot before bed (i.e., nurse both sides) when she starts sleeping for longer stretches at night, so be ready for that. She will gradually morph herself into a baby on a schedule. Follow her lead. As your baby develops her schedule, base it on her cues, not the clock. You'll get a feel for when she's tired, hungry, restless, and so forth. When your baby is older, then you will rely more on the clock.

Four Months: Your baby will be working toward a rough schedule at this point. It will look like this: baby wakes up (6:30 a.m.), then takes one morning nap (9:00 a.m. to 10:00 a.m.), one afternoon nap (1:00 p.m. to 3:00 p.m.), and one early evening nap (6:00 p.m. to 7:00 p.m.). The baby is sleeping at night (9:00 p.m.), only waking up to nurse (12:00 a.m., 4:00 a.m.) and have her diaper changed, and then falling back to sleep. Your baby still nurses on demand. Some babies forgo the evening nap and just go to bed earlier (7:00 p.m.) for the night. Mine never did that—but I know other babies who have. Let your little one set the bedtime at this age; you'll be able to tell from her signals. When she's crying, cranky, and fussy, she's tired and ready to sleep.

Six Months: You begin to feed your baby solid foods, introducing the concept of breakfast, lunch, and dinner into your baby's day. You still nurse on demand.

Nine Months: Your baby will lose the early evening nap by this time and will just have two naps during the day—morning and afternoon (for example, 9:00 a.m. and 2:00 p.m.). Your baby will wake with the family in the morning and go to bed around eight o'clock in the evening. This is the age I sleep trained my babies so they learned to sleep the entire night, without waking. I gave them a dream feed at ten o'clock, and, eventually, they didn't eat again until six o'clock in the morning. You can phase out the dream feed at eleven to twelve months. Mommy finally gets a good night's sleep! Yippee! During the day, Baby nurses a lot and is eating larger meals at mealtimes.

Twelve to Fifteen Months: Babies change from needing two naps to needing one nap a day around now. The best naptime for toddlers is directly after lunch (12:30 p.m. to 2:30 p.m. works well).

Bedtime Routine: Babies, toddlers, and young children all benefit from a regular and consistent bedtime routine. Here is ours:

> 6:30 p.m.: Bedtime snack
> 7:00 p.m.: Brush teeth, go pee, and bath time
> 7:30 p.m.: Put on pajamas and read bedtime stories
> 7:50 p.m.: Five minutes for kids to "read" in their beds with their lights on
> 7:55 p.m.: Lights out, hugs and kisses
> 8:00 p.m.: Sleeping

Of course, get ready for "I need a glass of water!" "I need to pee... again!" "I need a Band-Aid!" "My blankets fell off!" "I need an extra kiss!" "Sing me a lullaby...please!" Your kids will go through phases where they are more or less needy for your attention at bedtime. Be ready for their needs by having items on hand before your child asks.[164] "Good night, honey. Here is your tissue, Band-Aid, glass of water, extra kiss and hug, and blankie." If you follow your schedule and stay consistent, these needs and phases will be easier to manage. (They will come nonetheless! For example, one night I was nursing Maxwell, and I thought the other three were fast asleep like little angels when Terrek came in with a capless marker because he was worried the marker would

---

164 Susan Waite, mom

dry out. Then I heard Patrick calling from his bed, asking for more water. Then Evelyn crawled in my room on all fours saying, "I'm a puppy, I'm a puppy." Then Maxwell pooped.) Your schedule will come and will be specific to you and your kids. Sticking to it as best you can will help your sweet little ones carry out their days successfully and happily.

CHAPTER 38

Housekeeping Tips for Busy Moms and Dads

Why is there so much sand in the sink?

—ME

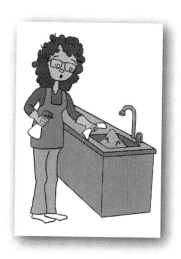

Did you think housekeeping was a chore before you had kids? Ha! The messiness of your house increases exponentially with the number of children you have. There are three reasons.

1. You have another person living in your house, making a mess.
2. With each additional person comes additional stuff.
3. You no longer have the time you used to have to devote to cleaning. Now your time is devoted to caring for your little one(s).

Your house will be messy. Sometimes I wonder if all kids are as messy as mine are. My kids seem to emit mud, crumbs, toys, dirty socks, milk spills, puddles, stickiness, and drips. There are two extremes of moms—the ones who don't care that their house is messy and keep on going. Great. Then there are the ones who can't stand a messy house because it drives them crazy! I was somewhere in the middle. I didn't mind toys all over the house as long as they were put away in their places and not scattered all over the floor. (We have bins, shelves, and toy areas in the kitchen, living, room, and dining room, but every toy has a spot where it belongs. What do you call that—organized chaos?) You might not know which kind of mom you are until you are actually a parent. Along the way, I have come across some great timesaving strategies to help you attempt to keep up with the house that somehow keeps messy-ing itself! (I don't recommend my husband's strategy for cleaning the table...with a vacuum—true story.)

- Get a housekeeper!
  - This is by far the best solution. It takes the pressure off you, it helps keep your sanity, and it buys you precious time to spend with your precious kids! However, it's expensive and not a reasonable option for most families (including mine). If you can afford it, do it!
  - Nannies can also help with housework when the kids are at school or napping. This is one invaluable asset of having a nanny.
- Get a robotic vacuum cleaner.[165]
  - These are small, handy, and much more affordable than a central vac. They work all by themselves and can be busy sucking up crumbs under the table while you're busy doing something else, like brushing everyone's teeth.
  - We love our iRobot Roomba, but the family member who loves it the most is my baby, Maxwell. He chases it around and squeals with delight when he sees it working. We've

---

165 Patricia Ryan, teacher and mom

had to hide it so he doesn't turn it on at random times during the day. He loves Roomba so much that I had his first birthday cake specially made in the shape of a Roomba. When he saw his cake, he signed "more, more" and attempted to press the button. ☺

- Teach your kids to pick up after themselves.
    - This is more difficult than one might think! It is a constant struggle—kids need training in this crucial habit and many reminders.
- Get your space organized.
    - Have labeled bins that are kid accessible, and train the kids to know where their toys go (cars, dolls, Mr. Potato Head, superheroes, etc.). When toys are all sorted like this, kids can more easily find what they're looking for—bonus!
    - Install hooks the kids can reach for their coats and backpacks, so they hang them up when they come in instead of throwing them on the floor.
    - Have cubbies for shoes, sunglasses, hats, scarves, and mitts. I find it most effective when each child has his own hooks and cubbies. Their belongings are always where they put them and not all mixed in with their siblings'.
- Switch to all-natural, nontoxic household cleaners. I have tried many different brands. Save money by using plain old vinegar and baking soda. They work just as well as cleaning products and are affordable and versatile. An added plus: they are edible and safe to inhale.
    - A ratio of one-third cup vinegar to two-thirds cup water in a spray bottle works well for mirrors, windows, and countertops.
    - Baking soda is great for toilets and sinks.
    - Make a paste of baking soda mixed with water and some all-natural dish soap (not regular dish soap, as that produces strong fumes when spread all around a surface, and you don't want to breathe them in). Use this to smear on tiles and the bathtub, then scour with a scrub brush or cloth, and rinse clean.

- o   Clean kitchen and bathroom floors with a bucket of warm water mixed with a few large glugs of vinegar.
- o   Wood floors and cupboards: simply wipe with a damp cloth.
- o   Note: baking soda and vinegar clean, but don't disinfect. I use a steamer for disinfecting.
- Keep baking soda and vinegar in the bathroom so you can spruce up your surfaces while your kids are taking a bath. While they are playing in the bubbles, squirt your mirror and sink, and scrub the toilet. This is multitasking at its finest. My kids always splish and splash so much that the floor gets pretty wet during a bath. When I wipe it up with a towel, the floor becomes dried and cleaned at the same time.
- Keep a table fan in the bathroom and turn it on after each shower/bath to prevent mold and mildew.
- Fold laundry while watching TV in the evening.
- Throw soap dishes, and bathroom cups in the dishwasher.[166]
- Keep each individual's laundry separate, so the laundry is always sorted even before it's done. (Each person gets his or her own hamper.) You eliminate the huge task of sorting and delivering laundry all over the house and save a whack of time.
  - o   Teach each person to put his dirty clothes in his own hamper in the closet.
  - o   Wash one load of clothes each day of the week so each person gets clean clothes once a week.
- Make a menu plan. Each week I plan meals for the following week and use this plan to create my grocery list. When it's time to make dinner, I'm never scrambling for what to make, and we're never missing ingredients.
- Give your kids some chores. As they get older, the breadth and depth of these tasks can increase, but start small (making bed, clearing plate, putting dirty laundry in the basket).
- Schedule your cleaning. Each day, complete one task, keeping it manageable so it doesn't become a huge chore on Saturday.

---

166 Patricia Ryan, teacher and mom

For example, Tuesday is bathroom day, and Thursday is vacuuming day.

- Get your ducts cleaned. This not only minimizes the need to dust around the house but also improves air quality so you and your baby can breathe easier. Be sure to hire a reputable company that actually does the work. If they charge ninety-nine dollars and are at your house for only one hour, it's a scam. Find a reputable, well-reviewed professional. Note: your house should never be dustier after they finish than before they started! See www.davesducts.com for guidelines; find a company near you that adheres to similar standards. The crew should be at your house for approximately three hours and should show you proof of his work, such as before-and-after photos from your ducts.[167]

While I love having a clean and organized house, it certainly isn't the most important thing. I always treasured the people in the house the most and the quality time we could spend together doing something fun and meaningful. However, the house is more enjoyable for the people who live there when it is organized and clean. Find the balance that works for you, and don't worry about what works for your neighbors or relatives. This is your life, your family, and your house!

167 www.davesducts.com

CHAPTER 39

A Note for Worrying Moms

Mommy! That is a flower 'gina. When I'm
big, will I grow flowers on my 'gina too?
—E., AGE THREE

I worry about my kids a lot. It started when I was pregnant, and it continues to this day. I worry that they will get hurt—are they safe? Are they eating healthy foods? Are they wearing their sunscreen? Does the sunscreen have harmful chemicals in it? Are they buckled up correctly? Does the bike helmet fit snugly? Should we get kneepads? Is our smoke detector functioning properly? Are they too hot? Are they too cold? Are they hydrated? Are they healthy? You can make yourself crazy with all the worrying. My husband used to say, "Relax! You're so anal." My response to him was always "I will not relax about my kids' safety, and yes, I'm anal, so get used to it. This is how I am." I have always believed that it is my job to keep my kids safe and to make sure they are OK. There is no such thing as being overprotective. It's just the right amount of protective! People say, "You can't keep them in a bubble." (Or can you? More on that later!) I agree that too much worrying can be counterproductive. But when moms worry about this, that, or the other thing happening to their child, and they think ahead, they actually do something to prevent said things from happening to their child. Then, that worrying was actually effective and had value after all!

I found it interesting to read recently in *MacLean's* magazine that mothers are genetically programmed to worry about their kids.[168] It is nature's way of ensuring the survival of the species. See? There is a purpose for our worrying. There should be studies on all the injuries and accidents that have been prevented because of a mom being proactive. If anyone bugs you about being "overprotective" of your kids, just say, "I can't help it; it's automatic. I'm just fulfilling my evolutionary responsibility."

As I said earlier, worrying can make you crazy. However, you are still going to do it. The unfortunate thing is that sometimes, you can worry so much that it stresses you out and then may have a negative effect on your health. If you are worrying about something that you have control over, turn your worry into action, and do something about it. If you are worrying about something that you have no control over, that is a waste of energy, and you need to find a way to deal with the concern. I have developed a few ways to help manage such stress and help maintain my sanity. Sometimes a song can help. I have two I turn to if I'm worrying about something I have no control over. "Que Sera Sera (Whatever Will Be, Will Be)," sung by Doris Day[169] ♪ and "Three Little Birds" (Don't Worry about a Thing) by Bob Marley and the Wailers.[170] ♪. Let yourself get lost in the music, and listen intently to the lyrics. It will help you settle your mind.

My second strategy is a little thought process/meditation I perform at night before I go to sleep. I relax, take a few deep breaths, and imagine I am like Bella from *The Twilight Saga*.[171] For those who haven't read it (you're missing out; go read the entire series right now! ☺), Bella is a vampire girl who can protect her family by emanating a protective force-field-type bubble from her body and engulfing her family in it. In my reverie, I imagine I can do the same thing. I

168 "The New Worry Epidemic," *Maclean's Magazine* (February 17, 2014), 56–59.

169 "Que Sera Sera (Whatever Will Be Will Be)," Doris Day, music by Jay Livingston, lyrics by Ray Evans, 1956.

170 "Three Little Birds," Bob Marley and the Wailers, *Exodus*, 1980, Tuff Gong.

171 Stephanie Meyer, *The Twilight Saga: Breaking Dawn* (New York: Little, Brown and Company; Hachette Book Group, 2008).

picture this bubble going around all my children, keeping them safe and healthy. Yes, maybe I sound crazy, but at least I can fall asleep believing that my kids are protected. While it may not actually "do" anything, it does work effectively to put my mind at ease and lets me go to sleep without worrying—and that is doing something!

CHAPTER 40

Rules at Our House

> Whatever I did…I did not do.
> —T., AGE SIX

1. Don't say "no" to Mommy.
2. No feet on faces.
3. Hands to yourself.
4. Sit down to eat.
5. No eating in the car.
6. No put-downs.
7. Treat one another nicely; we are kind to one another in our family.
8. Talk nicely; no whining.
9. Only write on paper (not on furniture, walls, people, etc. Terrek, my eldest, seemed to have great difficulty understanding this rule. He once drew a beard and mustache on his face with permanent marker and had to go to the dentist like that).
10. No running with sticks.
11. No wrestling near the baby.
12. Don't drink bathwater.
13. Say "sorry" if you hurt someone else (emotionally or physically).

CHAPTER 41

Top Ten Things You Never Thought You Would Enjoy before You Had Babies

> I want to touch Mommy's hair all day.
> —P., AGE THREE

10. Watching someone eat his or her vegetables.
9. Sitting in the scorching hot sun, watching kids play soccer, getting stung by a wasp while you fight to protect your kids from the same fate, while simultaneously getting goose poo all over your shoes.
8. The sweet silence when all little ones are finally asleep!
7. Finally finding the blankie you've spent the last forty minutes searching the house for so your little toddler can sleep.
6. The sweet sound of a burp.
5. Getting to "sleep in" until seven o'clock in the morning!
4. Being given a ripped and jagged scrap of paper with the sweet words, "I made this for you. It's a bracelet."
3. Your bed. (You've always enjoyed it, but you didn't know just how much you desperately love and miss your beautiful, soft, comfy bed.)
2. Witnessing successful pees and poos on the toilet that were not your own.
1. Being stared at all day by a bald person who drools.

CHAPTER 42

Other Useful Tips

> Man, I dropped my slug.
>
> —P., Age Four

- Keep a bag of clothes—one outfit per child—in the car. Remember to change it seasonally. Use a bag that zips so the clothes don't get dusty.
  - Note: don't keep the clothes in the back of the van by the wet/snowy stroller tires in the winter. I did that, and then when I needed them, as two out of four kids were sandy and soaked on an outing, I pulled out my bag of extra clothing. I was proudly appreciating myself for being such a prepared mom, when, to my unhappy surprise, I found the entire bag of clothing was damp and musty. My husband had to go to Walmart to buy new clothes for the wet and sandy kids. This plan tanked, but I am learning from my mistakes. Going forward, I will keep the bag of backup clothing in a nice, dry spot in the van and/or use a waterproof, tightly sealed bag!
- Stash extra diapers, Kleenex, and hand sanitizer in the car (we've forgotten our diaper bag on many occasions). If another baby is nearby, borrow from that family. Moms understand; we've all been there. Once we were up in the country without the diaper bag—no stores and no other babies anywhere. I had to improvise and use a pair of toddler underwear and a maxi pad, but hey—it worked!

- To check for a dirty diaper, simply lift baby up to your nose and smell the baby's bottom. You'll know right away whether it needs attention.
- After wiping your baby's face and hands with a wet cloth, be sure to dry your baby's face and hands with a dry cloth. Bacteria thrive in damp environments.[172] Many parents don't bother with this extra step, but I always do it so my baby is both clean and dry—it feels better to have a dry face.
- Keep your pinky fingernail long and your index fingernail short. Your pinky fingernail needs to be long so it can easily pluck out unwanted blockages from your tiny baby's nostrils.[173] Your index fingernail is best short so baby-bottom cream doesn't gum it up when you change a diaper.
- When strangers, random people and/or germy kids attempt to touch your vulnerable new born baby's face (believe me they will do it!), say politely: "please only touch her feet[174]." Once a complete stranger stroked Baby Patrick's chubby little cheeks when I was wearing him facing outward in my baby wrap. We were in a busy city market, and I had no idea what this woman's hands touched before they touched my baby's cheeks. Be ready for this!
- If your baby gets a scrape or small cut, and you can't put medi-cated ointment on it for fear he will eat it and/or get it in his eye, squirt some breast milk on the cut. Breast milk has natural antibiotic properties and can help prevent infection.[175]
- When Baby starts talking, keep a piece of paper on the fridge. Jot down all your baby's words and the age at which he said them. Write down the words the funny way he says them, and add them to his baby book later.
- Bring tablets or iPads to restaurants while your kids are tod-dlers and young children to keep them occupied so you can

---

172 Patricia Ryan, teacher and mom
173 Shalimar Santos-Comia, RN and mom
174 Ibid.
175 Ibid.

enjoy a meal out and have an adult conversation with your spouse. Ideally, you would teach your child to sit quietly and converse politely at a restaurant, but that is very difficult for a toddler, especially when there is more than one toddler! Have short conversations with the kids; then, when they begin to get crazy, whip out the tablets and let them play. Take the devices away when the food arrives and bring them back out when kids are finished eating. People will comment, "What well-behaved children you have. I could never take my toddlers out to dinner like that." This distraction also works for medical appointments.

- Develop a "patience mantra" for yourself. Heaven knows I have used mine many times! From the terrible twos to extreme dawdlers and school-age attitude, there have been many, many times when I felt ready to lose my cool. I would just breathe, and in my head—or even aloud, quietly—I would repeat "patience, patience." This helps me keep my cool and remember that I am dealing with a child. (Literally!)

- Needles at the doctor's office are always intimidating for toddlers and young kids. So when it's time to get that annual flu shot, the best thing to do is to let your kids have a lollipop. The trick is not to give the kids the lollipop after the shot is over; you need to let them begin licking the lollipop at precisely the same time they get the stick. The flavor distracts them from the pain. The trick works especially well if lollipops are a special treat they rarely—or even never—get, except for these occasions.

- I trained my kids to shout "alert" repeatedly if there was something that needed my immediate attention. If someone was stuck somewhere (e.g., climbed too high and couldn't get down), found something dangerous (e.g., a screw or broken glass), or if there was a big spill, I knew to come right away, and their siblings knew to watch out for whatever it was as well.

- Stock up on *lots* of Band-Aids. Toddlers and little children absolutely love Band-Aids. Evelyn and Maxwell like to wear them all the time for no reason. They even help (emotionally, that is) for bumps and bruises.

- No time for a facial? Just stick your head in the dishwasher midcycle for a warm steam treatment.
- *Always* pack snacks. Sometimes your kids may not eat them, but Murphy's Law will absolutely apply here—if you don't pack snacks, your kids will be starving and cranky. Case in point: one day at *Disney on Ice*, foolish me didn't pack snacks—I had just fed them before we left, and we were going to eat again directly after the show—tsk, tsk, Mommy! They were all starving. Daddy had to buy them very expensive pizza. ☺ Always pack snacks.
- Pots and pans can keep babies and toddlers entertained for a significant length of time!
- Buy organic fruits and vegetables, if possible, to minimize pesticide ingestion by your children. If organic is too expensive, at least wash your produce with a little bit of dish soap and rinse thoroughly.[176]
- When struggling to put on difficult baby/toddler shoes or boots (we're dealing with floppy, uncooperative feet here), focus on the heel. If you open the shoe/boot as wide as you can and concentrate on placing the baby's heel in the correct spot, the rest will follow.
- When putting on a shirt with a tight neck hole, develop the knack of getting it on or off quickly to minimize crying. You must fit it over Baby's huge noggin, fast. When putting such a shirt on, start with the crown (back top) of the head. Stretch the neck hole as large as you can and slip it over the crown first, then the face, and then the base of the head. When taking such a shirt off, bunch it up in your hands and slip it over Baby's face first. Then it comes right off. Babies want their eyes hidden by the shirt for the least amount of time possible.

---

176 Patricia Ryan, teacher and mom

- Keep your baby food jars. These are great for toddler-size drinking glasses and perfect for salad dressing in Mommy's and Daddy's packed lunches for work.
- Don't say "don't" to toddlers.[177] For instance, if you say, "Don't touch that!" they will touch it. If you say, "Don't eat that!" they will eat it. My mom's theory is that toddlers actually don't hear the word "don't" and think you are telling them to do exactly what you don't want them to do. This is especially true when you are shouting as if in a terrible rush because they are about to do something that could get them hurt, make them messy, or get them in some sort of trouble. Reword for better results. Instead of saying, "Don't play in the toilet!" say, "Touch the wall!" Instead of saying, "Don't jump off the stairs!" say, "Sit down!"
- Give your toddler a five-minute warning before you are about to leave somewhere. This will mentally prepare him for when it is actually time to go. When it is time to go, tell him to come. If he starts to have a fit, do not let him stay and play longer. Simply tell him it's time to go, and take him to the car, even if he's kicking and screaming!
- Sometimes moms have difficulty getting to sleep at night, or they wake up in the night, unable to get back to sleep. Often, we moms have too many things on our minds. "Don't forget to make an extra lunch for kid A. Kid B needs wart medicine. I need to write a teacher's note for kid C." The worry that you will forget things can interfere with a good night's sleep. Keep a notepad and pen beside your bed to jot these thoughts down and get them out of your head. You'll sleep better if you know they won't be forgotten. But if you don't have paper or are too tired to turn on your light, I have a trick for you! Remember my theory, of how actions facilitate learning? (See chapter 25, "Baby Sign Language.") It also applies for remembering. When I'm lying in bed, trying to sleep, and a worry or note to remember keeps circling my brain, and I do not

177 Ibid.

want to forget it, I make a physical gesture that represents this thought. For example, to pack a lunch, make the shape of a lunch box with your hands, then go to sleep. In the morning, you will remember the action, which will remind you of the thought. For me, it works every time.

- Keep a sense of humor. You may find yourself asking, "What's worse: my baby throwing up in my mouth or my seven-year-old son setting off the fire alarm at the grocery store?" (No, these things did not happen to me. They happened to my husband, which is why I can laugh about them. Just kidding. No, I'm actually serious. I do laugh about it.) It's all good! Keep a sense of humor!

CHAPTER 43

List of Funny Quotes from My Family Used in This Book

You have to admit, Mom, it's pretty funny.

—T., Age Eight

Note: keep a journal handy or use your smartphone to jot down funny things your children say and/or hilarious and completely strange things you find yourself saying. It's a way to help capture the magic of this stage in your life and keep your children forever young. Cue Rod Stewart![178] ♪

- "I need Mommy, or I'm going to collapse…I collapsed."—P., five
- "I don't like taking care of babies. It's too much work; they poo."—P., five
- "I sat on Patrick's dinner and Patrick sat on the bananas."—Me
- "Today, if the bananas fall off my pancake, I won't cry at all. Because I'm so excited about Christmas."—P., five
- "Maxwell, don't play with Terrek's penis. You have your own penis you can play with."—E., three
- "I don't like that song…it tastes weird."—E., three

---

178 "Forever Young," Rod Stewart, *Out of Order*, 1988, Warner Bros. Records.

- "I don't throw spoons. I'm big. I know what I'm doing."—E., three
- "Mommy, I love you harder than anything."—T., three
- "This is a picture of Mommy. This is her head, this is her hair, and these are her nipples."—P., four
- "It's going to be a girl? But we paid for a boy!"—T., four
- "When I was in your tummy, how did you know my name?"—T., four
- "Maxwell stole the butter and messed around with it when you were in the bathroom."—J., thirty-eight
- "Don't look at my privacy."—E., two
- (After dumping the entire crayon bucket and putting it on his head) "Hat."—M., one
- "When we were in your tummy, we played with your bellybutton."—T., four
- "Mommy, your nose is so big and pointy, it could cut a watermelon."—T., six
- "You're insane, like a duck."—P., five
- "I just landed on my butt-head."—E., three
- "Mommy, you'd better feed him now, with your nipples."—T., six
- "How can one mommy love one baby so incredibly much?"—Me
- "I need milk now, or else I'm going to get old."—P., four
- "I'm going to be a bad raccoon that likes everybody."—E., three
- "I'm so hungry. All that's in my tummy is only a speck, smaller than a germ."—P., four
- "Mommy, these peejamies are not working for me. They are making me not sleep." —E., three
- "Alert, alert, we've got a problem over here."—T., five
- "My tummy is hurt and I have a heck ache."—E., two
- "I want to stay with Mommy forever."—P., three
- "Why are there dead worms in my bed?"—Me
- "What about my stinky ear?"—P., four
- "Mommy, I have a tummy ache in my throat."—E., two

- "I found where the worms are coming from—from the boys' pockets."—Me
- "Me no like dresses. Bad pretty."—E., two
- "It's a good thing the squash exploded."—P., four
- "Mommy, I love you more than a crab."—P., three
- "Mommy, can you tuck me up?"—P., three
- "Ah! Maxwell coughed up a sticker!"—Me
- "I'm so thirsty. I haven't had milk in a year."—P., four
- "It's not my job to hold the bugs."—Me
- "Why are you crying?"—Me
  "Because Terrek is going to name me Ding-Dong."—P., four
- "This potty seat is broke. Nothing came out."—T., two
- "Don't want it. Don't like it. No wear it. I want my Spider-Man suit."—P., two
- "I'm the motor, but still, don't sit on my head, OK?"—P., four
- "Why is there so much sand in the sink?"—Me
- "Mommy! That is a flower 'gina. When I'm big, will I grow flowers on my 'gina too?" —E., three
- "Whatever I did...I did not do."—T., six
- "I want to touch Mommy's hair all day."—P., three
- "Man, I dropped my slug."—P., four
- "Can I go on a garbage truck when I'm an astronaut?"—T., four
- "In gym today, I looked at the sleeve of my pants, and I pulled out Maxwell's bib! I pushed it back in really fast because I didn't want everyone to see it!"—T., eight
- "Mommy, can you give me a leash for this cat? (Because it is a dog.)"—E., three
- "Mom! Mama! Mama! Mom!...Awesome."—M., one and a half

CHAPTER 44

Bun 2 Babe: The Soundtrack

> In gym today, I looked at the sleeve of my pants,
> and I pulled out Maxwell's bib! I pushed it back in
> really fast because I didn't want everyone to see it!
> —T., AGE EIGHT

♪ It really does seem too good to be true
  - "Can't Take My Eyes Off of You," Lauryn Hill, *The Miseducation of Lauryn Hill*, 1998, Ruffhouse Records & Columbia Records.

♪ You'll wish you had a million dollars
  - "If I Had a $1,000,000," The Barenaked Ladies, *Gordon*, 1993, Reprise Records.

♪ For now you're a shiny, happy person!
  - "Shiny Happy People," by R.E.M., *Out of Time*, 1991, Warner Bros. Records.

♪ You're so pregnant!
  - "I'm So Pregnant," Iggy Azalea "Fancy" Parody, written and produced by What's Up Moms, featuring Meg, vocals by Alyssa, rapping by Betsy, 2014. See https://www.youtube.com/watch?v=eVuittFyM34.

♪ Get ready to push…it
  - "Push It," Salt 'N Pepa, *Hot, Cool & Vicious*, released 1986, Next Plateau Records/London Records.

♪ Today is the greatest
  - "Today," Smashing Pumpkins, *Siamese Dream,* 1993, Virgin Records.

♪ Keep going, carry on
  - "Carry On," Fun., *One Night,* 2012, Ramen/Atlantic/Electra.

♪ Let's get it on
  - "Let's Get It On," Marvin Gaye, *Let's Get It On,* 1973, Tamla Records.

♪ You have a new pretty young thing to love
  - "P.Y.T. (Pretty Young Thing)," Michael Jackson, *Thriller,* 1983, Epic Records.

♪ This is the time to remember
  - "This Is the Time," Billy Joel, *The Bridge,* 1986, Columbia Records.

♪ Kiss your angel
  - "Lullabye (Goodnight, My Angel)," Billy Joel, *River of Dreams,* 1993, Columbia Records.

♪ Splish splash!
  - "Splish Splash," Bobby Darin, *Bobby Darin,* 1958, Atlantic Studios New York, Atco Records.

♪ It's a few hard days' nights
  - "Hard Day's Night," The Beatles, *Hard Day's Night,* 1964, EMI Studios, London, Label: Parlophone.

♪ Hey, Baby! Can't touch this!
  - "U Can't Touch This," M. C. Hammer, *Please, Hammer, Don't Hurt 'Em.* 1990, Capitol (US) Records.

♪ You must shake it off
  - "Shake It Off," Taylor Swift, *1989,* 2014, Big Machine Records.

♪When I'm worrying about something I have no control over…

- "Que Sera Sera (Whatever Will Be, Will Be)," Doris Day, music by Jay Livingston, lyrics by Ray Evans, 1956, Columbia Records.

♪Sometimes a song can help

- "Three Little Birds," Bob Marley and the Wailers, *Exodus*, 1980, Tuff Gong.

♪Capture the magic of this stage in your life and keep your children forever young… ♪Cue Rod Stewart!

- "Forever Young," Rod Stewart, *Out of Order*, 1988, Warner Bros. Records.

CHAPTER 45

Quoted Experts

> Mommy, can you give me a leash for
> this cat? (Because it is a dog.)
> —E., Age Three

- Dr. Karen Beal, chiropractor
- Howard Berger, MD, ob-gyn
- Dr. Lisa Doran, naturopathic doctor
- Claudette Leduc, registered midwife
- Ronald G. Morrish, parenting expert, educator, and behavior consultant
- Nadia Ramprasad, registered physiotherapist
- Rose Reyes, nanny
- Lisa Weston, registered midwife

Moms:

- Tamara Adamson, teacher and mom
- Maya Castle, mom
- Brenda Cuthbertson, mom
- Gerd Griffin, mom
- May Griffin, mom, grandmother, and great-grandmother of thirty-six children
- Oresta Korbutiak, mom
- Carolyn Lauchlan, mom

- Mary Miller, teacher and mom
- Amy Olar, teacher and mom
- Marian Orleans, mom
- Mary Anne Pangilinan, mom
- Charmayne Richards, teacher and mom
- Abigail Roberts, mom
- Patricia Ryan, teacher and mom
- Ellen Ryan-Chan, teacher and mom
- Shalimar Santos-Comia, nurse and mom
- Lisa Simms, mom
- Yvette Tsang, teacher and mom
- Susan Waite, mom

CHAPTER 46

References

> Mom! Mama! Mama! Mom!…Awesome.
> —M., Age One and A Half

Print

Cole, Joanna. *I'm a Big Sister*. New York: Harper Festival, 1997.

Harper, Barbara, RN, *Gentle Birth Choices.* Rochester, Vermont: Healing Arts Press, 2005.

Kingston, Anne. "The New Worry Epidemic." *Maclean's Magazine.* (February 17, 2014): 56–59.

Mayer, Mercer. *The New Baby*, New York: Random House, 1983.

Meyer, Stephanie. *The Twilight Saga: Breaking Dawn.* New York: Little, Brown and Company; Hachette Book Group USA, 2008.

Rapley, Gill, and Tracey Murkett. *Baby-Led Weaning.* London: Vermilion, 2008.

Ryan, Charlotte. "Creative Movement: A Powerful Strategy to Teach Science." MA diss., University of Toronto, 2006.

Websites

"ABC of Potty Training," Baby Center UK, accessed May 22, 2015, http://www.babycentre.co.uk/a4399/abc-of-potty-training.

"Blocked Ducts and Mastitis," Breastfeeding, Inc., accessed March 20, 2014, http://www.breastfeedinginc.ca/content.php?pagename=doc-BD-M.

"Breech Birth," Baby Center, accessed November 6, 2014, http://www.babycentre.co.uk/a158/breech-birth.

"Canada's Cord Blood System," Today's Parent, accessed August 17, 2015, www.todaysparent.com/pregnancy/giving-birth/canadas-cord-blood-system/.

"Car Seats: Information for Families for 2015," Healthychildren.org, accessed February 15, 2015, http://www.healthychildren.org/English/safety-prevention/on-the-go/Pages/Car-Safety-Seats-Information-for-Families.aspx.

"Child and Dependent Care Tax Credit," About Money, accessed May 22, 2015, http://taxes.about.com/od/deductionscredits/qt/child_care.htm.

"Childbirth in USA," Immihelp, accessed May 22, 2015, http://www.immihelp.com/nri/documents-after-childbirth-in-usa.html.

"Cursive Handwriting Is Disappearing from Public Schools," Washington Post, accessed May 22, 2015, http://www.washingtonpost.com/local/education/cursive-handwriting-disappearing-from-public-schools/2013/04/04/215862e0-7d23-11e2-a044-676856536b40_story.html.

"Diclectin for Morning Sickness," Motherisk, accessed May 16, 2015, http://www.motherisk.org/prof/updatesDetail.jsp?content_id=940.

"Does My Baby Need a Vitamin D Supplement?" Mayo Clinic, accessed August 18, 2015, www.mayoclinic.org/healthy-lifestyle/infant-and-toddler-health/expert-answers/vitamin-d-for-babies/faq-20058161.

"Does Vitamin B6 Help Relieve Morning Sickness?" Baby Center, accessed October 16, 2015, www.babycenter.com/404_does-vitamin-b6-help-relieve-morning-sickness_2519.bc.

"How Breastfeeding Benefits Mothers' Health," Scientific American, accessed March 20, 2014, http://www.scientificamerican.com/article/breastfeeding-benefits-mothers/.

"How Breastfeeding Benefits You and Your Baby," Baby Center, accessed March 2, 2014, http://www.babycenter.com/0_how-breastfeeding-benefits-you-and-your-baby_8910.bc.

"How Long Should My Baby Be in a Rear-Facing Car Seat?" The Globe and Mail Newspaper, accessed May 16, 2015,

http://www.theglobeandmail.com/globe-drive/culture/commuting/how-long-should-my-baby-be-in-a-rear-facing-car-seat/article5958964/.

"How Much Sleep Do Children Need?" WebMD, accessed June 5, 2015, http://www.webmd.com/parenting/guide/sleep-children.

"Is Dirt Good for Kids?" WebMD, accessed March 20, 2014, http://www.webmd.com/parenting/d2n-stopping-germs-12/kids-and-dirt-germs.

"Is It Safe to Eat Soft Cheese During Pregnancy?" Baby Center, accessed March 13, 2014, http://www.babycenter.com/404_is-it-safe-to-eat-soft-cheese-during-pregnancy_3175.bc.

"Is It Safe to Eat Sushi While Pregnant?" Baby Center, accessed March 13, 2014, http://www.babycenter.com/406_is-it-safe-to-eat-sushi-while-pregnant_1245280.bc.

iTunes: http://www.apple.com/ca/itunes/?cid=wwa-ca-kwg-music-itu, 02/25/2015.

"Mastitis, Causes," Mayo Clinic, accessed May 22, 2015, http://www.mayoclinic.org/diseases-conditions/mastitis/basics/causes/con-20026633.

"Maternity Leaves around the World: Worst and Best Countries for Paid Maternity Leave," Huffington Post, accessed May 16, 2015, http://www.huffingtonpost.ca/2012/05/22/maternity-leaves-around-the-world_n_1536120.html.

"Maternity Pay and Leave," Gov.UK, accessed May 16, 2015, https://www.gov.uk/maternity-pay-leave/leave."Midwife vs. OB-GYN, It Doesn't Have to Be a Competition," What to Expect, accessed May 16, 2015, http://www.what-toexpect.com/blogs/motherhoodloomswheresmyyarn/midwife-vs-obgyn-it-doesnt-have-to-be-a-competition.

"Miscarriage," Medline Plus, accessed May 31, 2015, http://www.nlm.nih.gov/medlineplus/ency/article/001488.htm.

"Mommy Brain," Today's Parent Magazine, accessed March 20, 2014, http://www.todaysparent.com/family/family health/mommy-brain/.

Motherisk: Motherisk Helpline: 1-877-439-2744, accessed May 22, 2015, http://www.motherisk.org/women/index.jsp.

"No Need to Delay Introduction of Food Allergens to High-Risk Babies," Canadian Pediatric Society, accessed March 20, 2014, http://www.cps.

ca/media/release-communique/no-need-to-delay-introduction-of-food-allergens-to-high-risk-babies.

"Postpartum Depression," Canadian Mental Health Association, accessed June 5, 2015, http://www.cmha.ca/mental_health/post-partum-depression/#.VXGrpFVVhHw.

"Rate of Infant Deaths in Unsafe Sleep Environments Unchanged Despite Increased Awareness: Ontario Coroner's Study," The Toronto Star Newspaper, accessed March 20, 2014, http://www.thestar.com/news/canada/2013/06/03/rate_of_infant_deaths_in_unsafe_sleep_environments_unchanged_despite_increased_awareness_ontario_coroners_study.html.

"Red Flags, Avoid Scammers, Here's How," Dave's Duct Cleaning, accessed February 16, 2015, www.davesducts.com.

Sesamestreet.org

"Should My Baby Wear Huggies?" The Green Lantern, Illuminating Answers to Environmental Questions, accessed August 26, 2015, http://www.slate.com/articles/health_and_science/the_green_lantern/2008/03/should_my_baby_wear_huggies.html.

"Signs Your Baby Has Gas and How to Treat It," Parents.com, accessed May 27, 2015, http://www.parents.com/baby/care/gas/signs-newborn-has-gas/.

Starfall.com

"Teeth: Dental Care for Children," About Kids' Health (From the Hospital for Sick Children) accessed May 22, 2015, http://www.aboutkidshealth.ca/En/HealthAZ/HealthandWellness/DentalCare/Pages/Teeth-Dental-Care.aspx.

"The Best Baby Sign Language Books," Start-American-Sign-Language, accessed March 20, 2014, http://www.start-american-sign-language.com/baby-sign-language-books.html.

"The Evidence for Doulas," Evidence-Based Birth, accessed May 22, 2015, http://evidencebasedbirth.com/the-evidence-for-doulas/.

"The Importance of Skin-to-Skin Contact," International Breastfeeding Centre, accessed March 20, 2014, http://www.nbci.ca/index.php?option=com_content&id=82:the-importance-of-skin-to-skin-contact-&Itemid=17.

"The Family Circus," The Family Circus Archives, accessed November 3, 2015, http://familycircus.com/strip-archives/.

"Toxoplasmosis," Wikipedia, accessed March 13, 2015, http://en.wikipedia.org/wiki/Toxoplasmosis.

"US Birth Certificates," Immihelp, accessed May 22, 2015, http://www.immihelp.com/nri/birthcertificate.html.

"Uterine Prolapse," US National Library of Medicine, National Institutes of Health, accessed August 23, 2015, http://www.ncbi.nlm.nih.gov/pmc/articles/PMC2034734/.

"Vaccines Do Not Cause Autism," Centre for Disease Control and Prevention, accessed July 17, 2014, http://www.cdc.gov/vaccinesafety/concerns/autism/.

"Wage and Hour Division, Family and Medical Leave Act," US Department of Labor, accessed May 16, 2015, http://www.dol.gov/whd/fmla/.

"What Is the Difference between Foremilk and Hindmilk?," La Leche League International, accessed March 20, 2014, https://www.llli.org/faq/foremilk.html.

Songs

For a complete list of all songs referenced in this book, see "Bun 2 Babe: The Soundtrack," *I listed the songs in order of appearance in the book.*

Lecture

Ronald G. Morrish, as heard in a parenting lecture, November 2011, Whitby, Ontario. Ronald Morrish is the author of *Secrets of Discipline* (Fonthill, Ontario: Woodstream Publishing, 1997).

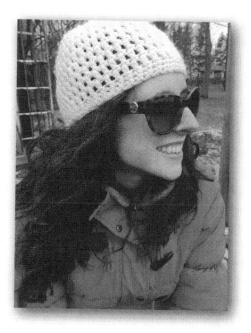

Charlotte Ryan, B.Sc. Hon., B.Ed., MA, is a special education teacher who earned her master's degree in education from the University of Toronto. She lives outside of Toronto with her husband and four wonderful children.

Made in the USA
Charleston, SC
15 March 2016